300
15-Minute
Low-Carb
Recipes

300
15-Minute
Low-Carb
Recipes

DELICIOUS MEALS THAT MAKE IT EASY TO LIVE YOUR LOW-CARB LIFESTYLE AND NEVER LOOK BACK

Dana Carpender

Author of *1001 LOW-CARB RECIPES*

FAIR WINDS
PRESS
BEVERLY, MASSACHUSETTS

Quarto is the authority on a wide range of topics.

Quarto educates, entertains and enriches the lives of
our readers—enthusiasts and lovers of hands-on living.

www.QuartoKnows.com

First published in the USA by
Fair Winds Press, an imprint of
Quarto Publishing Group USA Inc.
100 Cummings Center
Suite 406-L
Beverly, MA 01915-6101
Telephone: (978) 282-9590
Fax: (978) 283-2742
QuartoKnows.com
Visit our blogs at QuartoKnows.com

Library of Congress Cataloging-in-Publication Data available

19 18 17 16   7 8 9 10

ISBN-13: 978-1-59233-469-8
ISBN-10: 1-59233-469-5

Design by Leslie Haimes

Printed in the USA

In memory of the late Dr. Robert C. Atkins, 1930–2003.
Because of his fearless tenacity, millions of us live better lives today.

"If I can see far, it is because I have stood on the shoulders of giants."
—Sir Isaac Newton

contents

Introduction

Welcome to the world of *15~Minute Low Carb!*

I've known for a long time that, where cooking is concerned, I have a big edge over most of my readers. After all, I work at home. I can put something in the oven an hour or two before dinner and be here to tend to it if needed. I can simmer a pot of soup all afternoon. I'm here.

Furthermore, at this writing I have no children—only an exceedingly good-tempered and undemanding husband. In short, I never dash in the door at 6:15 p.m., after a long day at the office (and add a few errands on the way home into the bargain), to find people clamoring for me to get dinner on the table as soon as possible, and 5 minutes ago would be nice.

I also never slog home after a 12-hour day, so tired and hungry that the very idea of having to spend an hour getting dinner on the table is enough to send me through the local fast-food drive-in, even without a family to feed.

These are precisely the situations that this book is meant to help you cope with—all while keeping you on your low-carbohydrate diet and making your family happy.

Just What Do I Mean By 15 Minutes?

I mean exactly what I say—that from start to finish, these recipes take 15 minutes or less. I know this for certain because I set the stove timer when I started making them!

Now, it is entirely possible to make these dishes take a little bit longer. For instance, thawing times for frozen foods are not included, so if you haven't thought to take something out of the freezer in the morning, you'll just have to tack on however long it takes your microwave to thaw your food. (This would be a good time to sit down and have a glass of dry wine or a light beer, and maybe put out a tray of veggies and ranch dressing for the troops.) For that matter, more than once I've run two or three minutes over my time limit because I couldn't find the darned Worcestershire sauce or whatever. I take no responsibility for kitchen disorganization, and trust me, I know all about kitchen disorganization. However, once you have your ingredients located, the 15-minute count holds for these recipes, *prep time included.*

This, of course, rules out a fair number of dishes. You'll find no roasts in this book, no meat loaves—indeed, nothing that is cooked in an oven, because even if a dish requires less than 15 minutes in your oven, the preheating time is an obstacle. While there are wonderful soups, there are none of the traditional long-simmered variety. Indeed, you'll find that a few methods of cooking are used over and over, simply because they are speedy—sautéing, stir-frying, grilling, broiling, and microwaving.

You'll find that these recipes generally call for foods, especially meat and poultry, to be thinly cut, sliced, shredded, ground, or cubed. There's no mystery why: The smaller the pieces, the faster the cooking time! Thinly cut pork chops—about 1/4 inch (6 mm) thick—will cook within our time limit. Inch-thick (2.5 cm) pork chops, however, will not, no matter how juicy and delicious they may be. So if you're in doubt as you cut, chop, or slice your foods up, think "smaller is better."

You'll also find that these recipes call for you to multitask. Quite often I'll tell you to start one component of the dish cooking, then use that cooking time to cut up or measure and mix other ingredients. It's not hard, really—it's just making the best use of your time. Always give the directions a quick read before you go prepping everything in the ingredients list; you might find that there's a perfect time for chopping up veggies and the like without adding a second to your overall preparation and cooking time.

Low~Carb Menu Planning and One~Dish Meals

In the vast majority of the dishes in this book, the biggest source of carbo-hydrates is vegetables. I trust we can agree that this is the healthiest possible source of carbohydrates, no? Vegetables, however, are more than that—they are the most flavorful source of carbohydrates in our diet, and by cooking our very low-carb proteins with a variety of vegetables, we can create a widely varied, delicious, exciting low-carb cuisine. However, this will sometimes mean that your carbohydrate allowance for a given meal is completely used up by the vegetables in your soup or skillet supper. This, then, becomes a classic one-dish meal, and a beautiful thing it is.

What about My Carb-Eating Family?

No reason not to serve a carbohydrate food on the side, if your family will be bereft without it. However, I must say that many of the quickest, easiest carbohydrate side dishes—instant mashed potatoes, quick-cooking rice, whack-em-on-the-counter biscuits and rolls—are just as processed and nutrient-depleted as they can be and are also among the carbohydrates with the highest, most devastating blood sugar impact. Better to serve whole-wheat pita bread; corn or whole-wheat tortillas; one of the less damaging pastas (Jerusalem artichoke pasta, widely available at health food stores, has a relatively modest blood sugar impact and tastes like "regular" pasta); or potatoes you've cut into wedges, sprinkled with olive oil, and roasted in your toaster oven for about 15 minutes at 400°F (200°C, gas mark 6). If your family loves rice, well, brown rice is *hugely* superior to white rice, let alone Minute Rice, but it's nobody's idea of a 15-minute food. However, it reheats beautifully in the microwave. You could make a good-size pot of it over the weekend, stash it in the refrigerator, and use it later in the week. When you need it, just spoon out however much your family will need for the meal at hand, put it in a covered microwaveable container with a tablespoon (15 ml) or so of water, and nuke it on 70 percent power for a few minutes.

Anyway, the point is that if your family simply *insists* on a concentrated carbohydrate, serve it on the side. And because you love them, make it one of the less processed, less damaging carbohydrates.

What's a "Serving"?

I've gotten a couple of queries from folks who bought *500 Low-Carb Recipes* and want to know how big a serving size is, so I thought I'd better address the matter.

To be quite honest, folks, there's no great technical determination going on here. For the most part, a "serving" is based on what I think would make a reasonable portion, depending on the carbohydrate count, how rich the dish is, and for main dishes, the protein count. You just divide the dish up into however many portions the recipe says, and you can figure the carb counts on the recipes are accurate. In some cases I've given you a range —"3 or 4 servings," or whatever. In those cases, I've told you how many servings the carb counts are based on, and you can do a little quick mental estimating if, say, you're serving 4 people when I've given the count for 3.

Of course, this "serving" thing is flukey. People are different sizes and have different appetites. For all I know, you have three children under 5 who might reasonably split one adult-size portion. On the other hand, you might have one 17-year-old boy who's shot up from 5'5" to 6'3" in the past year, and what looks like 4 servings to me will be a quick snack for him. You'll just have to eyeball what fraction of the whole dish you're eating and go from there.

I've had a few people tell me they'd rather have specific serving sizes—like "1 cup" or the like. I see a few problems with this. First of all, it sure won't work with things like steak or chops—I'd have to use weights, instead, and then all my readers would have to run out and buy scales. Secondly, my recipes generally call for things like, "1/2 head cauliflower" or "2 stalks celery." These things vary in size a bit, and as a result yield will fluctuate a bit, too. Also, if one of my recipes calls for "1 1/2 pounds (680 g) boneless, skinless chicken breasts" and your package is labeled "1.65 pounds (750 g)," I don't expect you to whack off the difference to get the portions exact.

In short, I hate to have to weigh and measure everything, and I'm betting that a majority of my readers feel the same way, even if some do not. So I apologize to those who like exact measures, but this is how it's going to be for now, at any rate.

What's With the Info about Stuff other than Carbs and Protein?

You'll notice that in places in this book I've included notes regarding other nutritional components of some of the recipes. Most notably, I've included the calorie count if it seems quite low and the calcium or potassium count if it seems quite high. The reason for this is simple: Many people are trying to watch their calories as well as their carbs, and calling their attention to those dishes in this book that are particularly low in calories seemed helpful. Likewise, my e-mail tells me that the two nutrients low-carbers are most concerned they're *not* getting are calcium and potassium. So letting you know when a recipe is a good source of these nutrients also seemed helpful.

All of the recipes do, of course, include the carbohydrate, fiber, usable carbs, and protein counts.

On the Importance of Reading Labels

Do yourself a favor and get in the habit of reading the label on every food product, and I do mean every food product, that has one. I have learned from long, hard, repetitive experience that food processors can, will, and do put sugar, corn syrup, corn starch, and other nutritionally empty, carb-filled garbage into every conceivable food product. You will shave untold thousands of grams of carbohydrates off your intake over the course of a year by simply looking for the product that has *no added junk.*

There are also a good many classes of food products out there to which sugar is virtually always added—the cured meats immediately come to mind. There is almost always sugar in sausage, ham, bacon, hot dogs, liverwurst, and the like. You will look in vain for sugarless varieties of these products. However, you will find that there is quite a range of carb counts because some manufacturers add more sugar than others. I have seen ham that has 1 gram of carbohydrates per serving, and I have seen ham that has 6 grams of carbohydrates per serving—that's a 600 percent difference! Likewise, I've seen hot dogs that have 1 gram of carbohydrates apiece, and I've seen hot dogs that have 5 grams of carbohydrates apiece.

If you're in a position where you can't read the labels—for instance, at the deli counter at the grocery store—then ask questions. The nice deli folks will be glad to read the labels on the ham and salami for you, and they can tell you what goes into the various items they make themselves. You'll want to ask at the meat counter, too, if you're buying something they've mixed up themselves—Italian sausage, marinated meats, or whatever. I have found that if I state simply that I have a medical condition that requires that I be very careful about my diet—and I don't show up at the busiest hour of the week!—folks are generally very nice about this sort of thing.

In short, become a food sleuth. After all, you're paying your hard-earned money for this stuff, and it is quite literally going to become a part of you. Pay at least as much attention to your food shopping as you would if you were buying a car or a computer!

Appliances for 15-Minute Meals

There are a few kitchen appliances that you'll use over and over to make the recipes in this book. They're all quite common, and I feel safe in assuming that the majority of you have most, if not all, of these appliances.

A microwave oven. Surely everybody is clear by now on how quickly these both thaw and cook all sorts of things. We'll use your microwave over and over again to cook one part of a dish while another part is on the stove—to heat a broth, steam a vegetable, or cook the bacon that we're going to use as a topping.

It is assumed in these recipes that you have a microwave oven with a turntable; most of them have been made this way for quite a while now. If your microwave doesn't have a turntable, you'll have to interrupt whatever else you're doing and turn your food a few times during its microwaving time to avoid uneven cooking.

Also, be aware that microwaves vary in power, and my suggestions for power settings and times are therefore approximate. You'll learn pretty quickly whether your microwave is about the same power as mine or stronger or weaker.

One quick note about thawing things in the microwave: If you're coming home and pulling something right out of the freezer, you'll probably use the microwave to thaw it, and that's fine. However, if you can think of what you'd like to eat ahead of time, you can thaw in the fridge or even on the counter. (Wrap things in several layers of old newspaper if you're going to be gone for many hours and the day is warm. This will help keep things from going beyond thawing to spoiling.)

A good compromise is to thaw things most of the way in the microwave and then let them finish at room temperature. You retain more juices this way, but sometimes there's just no time for this.

A blender. You'll use this, or a stick blender, once in a while to puree something. You could probably use a food processor, instead. For that matter, while I use a standard-issue blender with a jar, there's no reason not to use one of those hand-held blenders.

A food processor. Chopping, grinding, and shredding ingredients by hand just doesn't fit into our time frame in many cases. If you don't yet own a food processor, a simple one that has an S-blade, plus a single disc that slices on one side and shreds on the other, shouldn't set you back more than $50 to $75.

An electric tabletop grill. Made popular by former Heavyweight Champion George Foreman, these appliances are everywhere. Mr. Foreman's version is quite good, but you can buy a cheaper version for all of 20 bucks. The burger chapter of this book assumes you have one of these appliances, but you can cook your burgers in a skillet instead or in some cases under the broiler. However, since these methods don't cook from both sides at once, you'll spend a few more minutes cooking this way than you would with the grill.

A slow cooker. What, I hear you cry, is a slow cooker doing in a book of *fast* recipes? Answering reader demand, that's what! I've gotten bunches of requests for slow cooker recipes from readers. Obviously, none of the slow cooker recipes will be done in 15 minutes. Instead, they require 15 minutes or less *prep time*, and that's including both the time to assemble the ingredients in the pot and the time to finish the dish and get it on the table when you get home.

If you don't have a slow cooker, consider picking one up. They're not expensive, and I see perfectly good ones all the time at thrift shops and yard sales for next to nothing. Keep your eyes open.

Techniques

There are just a few techniques that will help you get these recipes done in 15 minutes or less.

The Tilted Lid. Many of these recipes are cooked in a skillet. Covering the skillet will speed up cooking, but it also holds in moisture, which is not always what we want. Therefore, I sometimes use the "tilted lid" technique: I put the lid on the skillet but tilt it slightly to one side, leaving about a 1/2-inch (1.3 cm) gap. This allows steam to escape, while still holding some heat in the pan. When I refer in a recipe to putting a "tilted lid" on the pan, this is what I mean. This is a good technique to use any time you want to speed up a skillet recipe without holding in moisture.

Pounding Meat. It takes only a half a minute or so to beat a boneless, skinless chicken breast or a piece of pork loin until it's 1/2- to 1/4- (13 to 6 mm) inch thick all over, and it cuts a good 5 to 10 minutes off the cooking time—a worthwhile tradeoff. Pounding meat is very easy to do. You just put your chicken breast or piece of pork loin or whatever in a heavy zipper-lock plastic bag, press out the air, and seal it. Then, using any heavy object—a hammer, a dumbbell, or an actual meat-pounding device—you pound the sucker all over with barely controlled ferocity (you want to use a tiny bit of control, or you'll pound right through it) until it's a thin sheet of meat. This technique also tenderizes the meat nicely. Once you've done this a time or two, you'll wonder why you haven't been doing it all along.

Guar or Xanthan Shaker. You'll find a description of these ingredients a little further on—they're thickeners, and they're very useful for replacing flour and cornstarch in gravies and sauces.

In *500 Low-Carb Recipes*, I recommended always putting guar or xanthan through your blender with part of the liquid to be thickened, so you could avoid lumps. You may now happily forget that technique. Instead, acquire an extra salt shaker and fill it with guar or xanthan. This will live next to your stove. Whenever you want to thicken a dish, simply sprinkle guar or xanthan over the top of the dish to be thickened, a little at a time, stirring madly all the while (preferably with a whisk). Stop when the dish is just a little less thick than you'd like it to be, as these thickeners will thicken a little more on standing. This works nicely, is worlds easier than transferring stuff into the blender, and doesn't leave you with a blender to wash!

Ice Cube Preservation. This isn't a cooking technique, it's a money-saving technique. A lot of these recipes call for small quantities of things which, in large quantities, would make the dish too high-carb for us—1/2 cup (123 g) of spaghetti sauce, 1/4 cup (60 g) of canned crushed pineapple, 2 tablespoons (32 g) of tomato paste, that sort of thing. I don't know about you, but I'm not about to let the leftovers of those ingredients grow fur in the back of my fridge, only to be thrown away. So I spoon the remainder of the contents into ice cube trays, freeze the resulting spaghetti sauce cubes or pineapple cubes or whatever, pop 'em out, and store 'em in zipper-lock bags in the freezer. That way, the next time I want to use that ingredient, I can thaw just the little bit I need.

Convenience Foods

In this book, I have made more liberal use of convenience foods than I normally do. As to the availability of these ingredients, I figured if I could get it in Bloomington, Indiana—a southern Indiana town of 65,000 people—it would be available to a majority of my readers, at least in the United States. You will find that these recipes call for all of the following.

Bagged salad. Where in *500 Low-Carb Recipes* I would have told you to shred half a head of cabbage, in this book I tell you to use bagged coleslaw mix.

Instead of washing fresh spinach (which can often take three or four washings), I've used bagged baby or triple-washed spinach. Mixed greens, European blends—all kinds of bagged salads show up in this book.

Bottled salad dressings. I've used bottled vinaigrette, ranch, Italian, blue cheese, and Caesar dressings in these recipes. These varieties of salad dressings are pretty reliably low-carb, but read the labels to find the brand with the lowest carb count. And this may be just my bias, but I think Paul Newman's salad dressings are excellent.

Chili garlic paste. This is actually a traditional Asian ingredient, consisting mostly, as the name strongly implies, of hot chilies and garlic. This seasoning saves lots of time when we want a recipe to be both hotly spicy and garlicky. Chili garlic paste comes in jars and keeps for months in the refrigerator. It's worth seeking out at Asian markets or particularly comprehensive grocery stores.

Crushed pork rinds. You can make crushed pork rinds very easily: Simply pour a bag of pork rinds into your food processor with the S-blade in place and run it until you have something the consistency of bread crumbs. Store in a tightly closed container in the refrigerator. I like to have both plain and barbecue-flavor crushed pork rinds on hand.

Frozen vegetables. Because they're already prepped and ready to go, frozen vegetables save a great deal of time in some of these recipes—for instance, trimming and cutting up green beans would take up most of our 15-minute time limit, while you can pour a bag of frozen green beans into a microwaveable container and start them cooking in less than a minute.

I've also used some vegetable blends in this book. This is a great way to get a variety of vegetables in a dish with no extra work.

Jarred Alfredo sauce. This is a nice ingredient for making simple meat and vegetables into a skillet supper, and it's usually lower carb than tomato-based spaghetti sauce. Read your labels, of course, to find the lowest-carbohydrate brand.

Jarred, grated gingerroot. Grated gingerroot is an extraordinary spice. Dried, ground ginger is no substitute, and for this reason I have long kept a gingerroot in a zipper-lock bag in my freezer, ever-ready for grating or mincing. However, this does take at least a few precious minutes. Fortunately, grated gingerroot in oil, put up in jars, is now widely available. I have used this prepared grated gingerroot in testing these recipes and like it so much that I may keep on using it now that this book is done!

If you can't find grated gingerroot in jars, I see no reason not to buy a fresh gingerroot, peel it, run it through the shredding blade of your food processor, are then chop the resulting shreds still further with your S-blade. (Don't grate up more gingerroot than you can use in a few weeks, though; it's best when it's fresh.) Spoon the resulting paste into a jar with a tight lid, add enough canola, peanut, or sunflower oil to cover, and store in the fridge. This will give you grated gingerroot at your fingertips.

Jarred minced garlic. Truth to tell, I greatly prefer fresh garlic, freshly crushed, over any possible substitute. But jarred, minced garlic in oil is very popular and widely available—and it is, no doubt, quicker than crushing fresh garlic, by at least a minute or two. Therefore, I have used jarred, minced garlic in these recipes. I have, however, always given the equivalent measure of fresh garlic, should you, like me, prefer it enough to be willing to take the extra few seconds.

Low-carbohydrate tortillas. La Tortilla Factory makes these, and they're becoming easier and easier to find—I know of at least a few stores here in Bloomington that carry them. (For you locals, they include Bloomingfoods, Marsh, and Kroger.) If you can't find these locally, you could ask your local health food store to special-order them for you. There are also a reasonable number of "e-tailers"—online retailers—who offer these.

Low-sugar or no-sugar barbecue sauce and ketchup. There are a number of these on the market; look around or check the e-tailers. However, I have also included recipes for both of these in the *Condiments, Sauces, Dressings, and Seasonings* chapter of this book (see page 289). They're very useful to have on hand.

Low-sugar preserves. In particular, I find low-sugar apricot preserves to be a wonderfully versatile ingredient. I buy Smucker's brand, and I like it very much. This is lower in sugar by *far* than "all fruit" preserves, which replace sugar with concentrated fruit juice. Folks, sugar from fruit juice is still sugar.

Smucker's also makes artificially sweetened preserves, but they only have about 1 fewer gram of carbohydrates per serving than the low-sugar variety, and many people prefer to avoid aspartame, so I use the low-sugar variety.

Shredded cheese. Virtually every grocery store in America carries shredded cheddar, Monterey Jack, mozzarella, Mexican blend, and the like. When this book calls for shredded cheese, I'm assuming you bought it that way. I'm also assuming that if a recipe calls for crumbled blue cheese, you bought it crumbled.

Sliced mushrooms. A couple of years ago I discovered that my local grocery stores had started selling fresh mushrooms already sliced for the same price as unsliced mushrooms. I never looked back! Whenever a recipe calls for sliced mushrooms, I'm assuming that you bought them already sliced.

Sprinkle-on seasoning blends. There are some recipes for these in the *Condiments, Sauces, Dressings, and Seasonings* chapter (see page 289), but I've also used some store-bought seasoning blends, all of which are widely available—lemon pepper, Old Bay seasoning, Creole seasoning, barbecue dry-rub seasoning (sometimes called "soul" seasoning), and a wonderful Rosemary-Ginger Rub from Stubb's, of Austin Texas. (Indeed, everything from Stubb's is great, and every product of theirs that I've tried has been lower in sugar than the run-of-the-mill.)

Tapenade. Tapenade is a wonderful relish or spread made mostly of chopped olives. While it's traditionally spread on bread, it adds an exciting flavor to several recipes in this book but saves you the work of chopping up olives, onions, and various other things. Look for tapenade in jars in your grocery store—it will usually be with the olives and pickles, but it might be in the International section, instead.

Basic Ingredients

These are some ingredients I consider standards for low-carb cooking in general—those of you who have read *500 Low-Carb Recipes* may notice these descriptions are familiar.

Avocados. Several recipes in this book call for avocados. Be aware that the little, black, rough-skinned avocados are far lower in carbohydrates (and higher in healthy monounsaturated fat) than the big green ones. All nutritional analyses were done assuming you used little black avocados.

Beer. One or two recipes in this book call for beer. The lowest carbohydrate beers on the market at this writing are Bud Select 55 (1.9 g carb) and Miller Genuine Draft Light 64 (MGD 64) (2.4 g carb). These are what I recommend you use. They are also what I recommend you drink, if you're a beer fan.

Blackstrap molasses. What the heck is molasses doing in a low-carb cookbook? It's practically all carbohydrates, after all! Well yes, but I've found that combining Splenda with a very small amount of molasses gives a good, brown-sugar flavor to all sorts of recipes. Always use the darkest molasses you can find—the darker it is, the stronger the flavor and the lower the carb count. That's why I specify blackstrap, the darkest, strongest molasses there is. It's nice to know that blackstrap is also where all the minerals they take out of sugar end up—it may be carby, but at least it's not a nutritional wasteland. Still, I only use small amounts. It's easiest to measure these small quantities if you store your blackstrap in a squeeze bottle—mine is in one of those plastic "honey bears."

You may be asking why I don't just use some of the artificial brown-sugar flavored sweeteners out there. The answer is because I've tried them, and I haven't tasted a one I would be willing to buy again. Ick.

Bouillon or broth concentrates. Bouillon or broth concentrate comes in cube, crystal, or liquid form. It is generally full of salt and chemicals and doesn't taste notably like the animal it supposedly came from. It definitely does *not* make a suitable substitute for good-quality broth if you're making a pot of soup. However, these products can be useful for adding a little kick of flavor here and there—more as seasonings than as soups—and for this use, I keep them on hand. I generally use chicken bouillon crystals because I find them easier to use than cubes. I also keep liquid beef broth concentrate on hand. I chose this because, unlike the cubes or crystals, it actually has a bit of beef in it. I use Wyler's, but I see no reason why any comparable product wouldn't work fine. If you can get the British product Bovril, it's probably even better! Since first writing this, I have discovered Better Than Boullion, which is the best product of this kind I've tried. It is now my standard.

Fish sauce. Called nuoc mam in Vietnam and nam pla in Thailand, this is a salty, fermented seasoning widely used in Southeast Asian cooking. It's available in Asian grocery stores and in the Asian foods section of big grocery stores. Grab it when you find it; it keeps nicely without refrigeration. Fish sauce is used in a few really great recipes in this book, and it adds an authentic flavor. In a pinch, you can substitute soy sauce, although you'll lose some of your Southeast Asian accent.

By the way, fish sauce is not the same thing as Chinese oyster sauce.

Guar and xanthan. These sound just dreadful, don't they? But they're in lots of your favorite processed foods, so how bad can they be? You're probably wondering what the heck they are, though. They're forms of water-soluble fiber, extracted and purified. Guar and xanthan are both flavorless white powders; their value to us is as low-carb thickeners. Technically speaking, these are carbs, but they're all fiber—nothing but. So don't worry about it.

Your health food store may be able to order guar or xanthan for you—I slightly prefer xanthan, myself—if they don't have them on hand. You can also find it online. Keep either one in a jar with a tight lid, and it will never go bad. I bought a pound of guar about 15 years ago and it's still going strong!

Low-carbohydrate bake mix. There are a few brands of low-carbohydrate bake mix on the market. These are generally a combination of some form of powdery protein and/or fiber—soy, whey, sometimes oat—plus baking powder and sometimes salt. These are the low-carb world's equivalent of Bisquick, although low-carb bake mixes differ from Bisquick in that they do not have shortening added. You will need to add butter, oil, or some other form of fat when using these mixes to make pancakes, waffles, biscuits, and the like. I mostly use low-carb bake mix in lesser quantities for things like "flouring" chicken before baking or frying or for making batter to fry onion rings in. If you can't find lit locally, there are many websites that sell it.

Bland oils. Sometimes you want to use a bland oil in a recipe—something that adds little or no flavor of its own. In this case, I recommend peanut, sunflower, or canola oil. These are the oils I mean when I simply say "oil." Avoid highly polyunsaturated oils such as safflower oil; they deteriorate quickly both from heat and from contact with oxygen, and they have been associated with an increased risk of cancer.

Olive oil. It surely will come as no surprise to you that olive oil is a healthy fat, but you may not know that there are various kinds. Extra-virgin olive oil is the first pressing. It is deep green, with a full, fruity flavor, and it makes all the difference in salad dressings. However, it is expensive and it's too strongly flavored for some uses. I keep a bottle of extra virgin olive oil on hand, but I use it exclusively for salads.

For sautéing and other general use, I use a grade of olive oil known as "pomace." Pomace is far cheaper than extra-virgin olive oil and has a milder flavor. I buy pomace in gallon cans at a local grocery specializing in Mediterranean foods. These gallon cans are worth looking for; it's the cheapest way to buy the stuff. If you can't find gallon cans of pomace, feel free to buy whatever cheaper, milder-flavored olive oil is available in your grocery store.

Be aware that if you refrigerate olive oil it will become solid. This is no big deal; it will be fine once it warms up again. If you need it quickly, you can run the bottle under warm water or microwave it for a minute or so on low power (assuming the container has no metal and will fit in your microwave).

Onions. Onions are a borderline vegetable; they're certainly higher in carbohydrates than, say, lettuce or cucumbers. However, they're loaded with valuable phytochemicals, so they're very healthful, and of course they add an unmatched flavor to all sorts of foods. Therefore I use onions a lot, but I try to use the least quantity that will give the desired flavor. Indeed, one of the most common things I do to cut carb counts on "borrowed" recipes is to cut back on the amount of onion used. If you have serious diabetes, you'll want to watch your quantities of onions pretty carefully and maybe even cut back further on the amounts I've given.

If you're not an accomplished cook, you need to know that different types of onions are good for different things. There are mild onions, which are best used raw, and there are stronger onions, which are what you want if you're going to be cooking with them. My favorite mild onions are sweet red onions; these are widely available, and you'll see that I've used them quite a lot in the recipes. However, if you prefer, you can substitute Vidalia or Bermuda onions anywhere I've specified sweet red onions. Scallions, also known as green onions, also are mild and are best eaten raw or quickly cooked in stir-fries. To me, scallions have their own flavor, and I generally don't substitute for them, but your kitchen won't blow up or anything if you use another sort of sweet onion in their place.

When a recipe simply says "onion," what I'm talking about is good old yellow globe onions, the ones you can buy in net sacks. You'll be doing yourself a favor if you pick a sack with smallish onions in it—that way, when a recipe calls for just 1/4 or 1/2 cup (40 to 80 g) of chopped onion, you're unlikely to be left with half an onion on your hands. For the record, when I say simply, "a small onion" I mean one about 1 1/2 inches (3.8 cm) in diameter, or about 1/4 to 1/3 cup (40 to 53 g) when chopped. A medium onion would be about 2 inches (5 cm) in diameter and would yield between 1/2 and 3/4 cup (80 and 120 g) when chopped. A large onion would be 2 1/2 to 3 inches (6.4 to 7.5 cm) across and will yield about 1 cup (160 g) when chopped. Personally, I'm not so obsessive about exact carb counts that I bother to measure every scrap of onion I put in a dish; I think in terms of small, medium, and large onions, instead. But that's up to you.

Packaged broths. Canned or boxed chicken broth and beef broth are very handy items to keep around, and they're certainly quicker than making your own. However, the quality of most of the canned broth you'll find at your local grocery store is appallingly bad. The chicken broth has all sorts of chemicals in it and often sugar, as well. The "beef" broth is worse—it frequently has no beef in it whatsoever. I refuse to use the majority of these products, and you should, too.

However, there are a few canned or boxed broths on the market worth buying. Many grocery stores now carry a brand called Kitchen Basics, which contains no chemicals at all. It is packaged in quart-size boxes (one litre in the UK), much like soy milk. Kitchen Basics comes in both chicken and beef. Health food stores also have good-quality canned and boxed broths—both Shelton and Health Valley brands are widely distributed in the United States.

Decent packaged broth will cost you a little more than the stuff that is made of salt and chemicals, but not a whole lot more. If you watch for sales, you can often get it as cheaply as the bad stuff and stock up. When my health food store runs a sale on good broth, I buy piles of the stuff!

One last note—you will also find canned vegetable broth, particularly at health food stores. This is tasty, but it runs much higher in carbohydrates than the chicken and beef broths. I'd avoid it.

Rice protein powder. For use in savory recipes—entrées and such—you need protein powder that isn't sweet, and preferably one that has no flavor at all. There are a number of these on the market, and some are blander than others. I've tried several kinds, and I've found that rice protein powder is the one I like best. I buy Nutribiotic brand, which has 1 gram of carbohydrates per tablespoon (10 g), but any unflavored rice protein powder with a similar carb count should work fine. For that matter, I see no reason not to experiment with other unflavored protein powders, if you like. If you can't find rice protein powder, ask your local health food store to order it for you—most health food stores are lovely about special orders.

Sucralose. I'm a fan of sucralose, aka Splenda. I think it tastes great. Splenda is the latest artificial sweetener to hit the market, and it blows all of the competition clear out of the water! Feed nondieting friends and family Splenda-sweetened desserts and they will never know that you didn't use sugar. It tastes that good.

Splenda has some other advantages. The table sweetener has been bulked so that it measures spoon-for-spoon and cup-for-cup just like sugar. This makes adapting recipes much easier. Also, Splenda stands up to heat, unlike aspartame, which means you can use it in baked goods.

However, Splenda is *not* completely carb-free. Because of the malto-dextrin used to bulk it, Splenda has about 0.5 gram of carbohydrate per teaspoon, or about one eighth of the carbohydrates of sugar. So count 0.5 gram per teaspoon, 1 1/2 grams per tablespoon (0.5 g), and 24 grams per cup (25 g). At this writing, MacNeill, the company that makes Splenda, has no plans to release liquid Splenda in the United States, but I am hoping that they will change their minds. The liquid, available in some foreign countries, is carb-free, and while it will take a little more finesse to figure out quantities, it will allow me to slash the carb counts of all sorts of recipes still further.

Tomatoes and tomato products. Tomatoes are a borderline vegetable, but they are so nutritious, flavorful, and versatile that I'm reluctant to leave them out of low-carb cuisine entirely. After all, lycopene, the pigment that makes tomatoes red, has been shown to be a potent cancer-fighter. Who wants to miss out on something like that?

You'll notice that I call for canned tomatoes in a fair number of recipes, even some where fresh tomatoes might do. This is because fresh tomatoes aren't very good for much of the year, while canned tomatoes are all canned at the height of ripeness. I'd rather have a good canned tomato in my sauce or soup than a mediocre fresh one. Since canned tomatoes are generally used with all the liquid that's in the can, the nutritional content doesn't suffer the way it does with most canned vegetables.

Canned diced tomatoes with green chilies have become widely available in the past few years, and what a welcome addition they are! They let us add two great flavors by opening just one can.

I also use plain canned tomato sauce, canned pizza sauce, canned pasta sauce, and jarred salsa. When choosing these products, you need to be aware that tomatoes, for some reason, inspire food packers to flights of sugar-fancy. They add sugar, corn syrup, and other carb-laden sweeteners to all sorts of tomato products. So it is even more important that you read the labels on all tomato-based products to find the ones with no added sugar. And keep on reading them! The good, cheap brand of salsa I used for quite a while showed up one day with "New, Improved!" on the label. Guess how they'd improved it? Right. They'd added sugar. So I found a new brand.

Vege-Sal. If you've read my newsletter, *Lowcarbezine!*, you know that I'm a big fan of Vege-Sal. What is Vege-Sal? It's a salt that's been seasoned, but don't think "seasoned salt." Vege-Sal is much milder than traditional seasoned salt. It's simply salt that's been blended with some dried, powdered vegetables. The flavor is quite subtle, but I think it improves all sorts of things. I've given you the choice between using regular salt or Vege-Sal in a wide variety of recipes. Don't worry, they'll all come out fine with plain old salt, but I do think Vege-Sal adds a little something extra. Vege-Sal is also excellent sprinkled over chops and steaks in place of regular salt. Vege-Sal is made by Modern Products and is widely available in health food stores.

Vinegar. Various recipes in this book call for wine vinegar, cider vinegar, rice vinegar, tarragon vinegar, white vinegar, and balsamic vinegar. If you've always thought that vinegar was just vinegar, think again! Each of these vinegars has a distinct flavor all its own, and if you substitute one for the other, you'll change the whole character of the recipe—one splash of cider vinegar in your Asian Chicken Salad, and you've traded your Chinese accent for an American twang. Vinegar is such a great way to give bright flavors to foods while adding few carbs that I keep all of these varieties on hand—it's not like they go bad or anything.

As with everything else, read the labels on your vinegar. I've seen cider vinegar that has 0 grams of carbohydrates per ounce, and I've seen cider vinegar that has 4 grams of carbohydrates per ounce—that's a huge difference! Beware, also, of apple cider *flavored* vinegar—white vinegar with artificial flavors added. I bought this once by mistake, so I thought I'd give you the heads-up. (You'd think the Label Reading Police would be beyond such errors, wouldn't you?)

Wine. There are several recipes in this cookbook calling for either dry red or dry white wine. I find the inexpensive wines that come in a mylar bag inside a cardboard box to be very convenient to keep on hand for cooking for the simple reason that they do not go bad because the contents are never exposed to air. These are not fabulous vintage wines, but they're fine for our modest purposes, and they certainly are handy. I generally have both Burgundy and Chablis box wines on hand. Be wary of any wine with "added flavors"—too often, one of those flavors will be sugar. Buy wine with a recognizable name—Burgundy, Rhine, Chablis, Cabernet, and the like, rather than stuff like "Chillable Red."

Coconut Flour. Once the coconut oil is pressed out of coconut meat, the remaining mass is finely ground into coconut flour. The stuff is loaded with fiber: 2 tablespoons (16 g) have 10 grams of carbohydrate, of which 6 grams are fiber. It has 2 grams of protein, too. There's a real learning curve to cooking with coconut flour because of the super-high fiber content; the stuff sucks up moisture in baking recipes. But in this book, we primarily use it to flour poultry or fish, which is far less problematic. Around here, Bob's Red Mill brand coconut flour is pretty widely available; I've seen it in health food stores and regular grocery stores, both. If you can't find coconut flour in stores near you, CarbSmart.com and Amazon.com both carry it.

Coconut oil. Long shunned because of its very high content of saturated fat, coconut oil has emerged as one of the healthiest fats you can use. I can now find it with the other oils at my local Kroger, or you can find it at health food stores and Asian markets. Whether your coconut oil smells and tastes like coconut depends on the brand; I've found that the expensive extra-virgin coconut oil has a coconut fragrance, while the inexpensive stuff is quite bland. Don't bother refrigerating coconut oil—because of its saturation it is extremely stable and won't go rancid on you.

Sriracha. This is Southeast Asian hot sauce, and it's taking over the world—*Bon Appetit* magazine declared it The Ingredient of the Year. Find Sriracha in the international aisle of big grocery stores or in Asian markets— look for the bright-red sauce with the rooster on the bottle.

Erythritol. This is one of the polyol or sugar alcohol sweeteners and the one I use most often. Unlike maltitol, which is widely used in commercial sugar-free sweets, erythritol has very little gastrointestinal effect. It also has the lowest absorption profile of all the sugar alcohols, so it has virtually no usable carbohydrate, while I generally count half a gram for maltitol. My local health food stores all carry erythritol, but again, you can buy it through CarbSmart. com or Amazon.com if you can't find it locally.

Granular Sucralose. Since *15 Minute Low-Carb Recipes* was first published, sucralose, best known by the trade name Splenda, has gone off-patent. There are now dozens of knock-offs and store brands, and there's no reason not to use them instead of the name brand. Do look for one that measures cup-for-cup like sugar. Be wary of brown sugar blends and other sucralose blends; these have sugar in them. And remember that because of the malto-dextrin used to bulk it, granular sucralose has about 24 grams of carbohydrate per cup—the 0 carb figure is an artifact of the teeny serving size listed on the label.

Liquid Sucralose. More and more I use liquid sucralose because it's carb-free. I use EZ Sweetz brand, which I buy in dropper bottles from Amazon.com; one drop is the equivalent of 2 teaspoons of sugar—or granular sucralose—in sweetness. I have also heard good things about Sweetzfree brand. If you buy liquid sucralose, read the label of whichever brand you buy to work out the equivalencies to sugar/granular sucralose.

Sugar-Free Coffee Flavoring Syrups. I specify *coffee flavoring* not because they're only useful for flavoring coffee—indeed, some flavors, like pineapple, would be wretched in coffee. Rather, I want to differentiate these from stuff like sugar-free Hershey's Syrup or pancake syrup. I'm talking about the sort of syrups you would find in a fancy coffee shop—vanilla, caramel, hazelnut, etc. A modest collection of these syrups broadens your culinary horizons considerably, especially if you like smoothies. The most widely available brands are DaVinci, Torani, and Monin's—they're all good. If you can't find them locally, they're available online.

Tofu Shirataki. Finally, there's a genuinely low carb noodle! Shirataki are a traditional Japanese noodle made from a root called kojac or *konyaku*, sometimes mistakenly translated **yam** or **yam bean**. The konjac root is a rich source of a fiber called glucomannan, and it is that glucomannan fiber that forms the bulk of shirataki noodles.

Shirataki come in two basic varieties. There is traditional shirataki and tofu shirataki. Traditional shirataki are translucent and gelatinous and very . . . well, Asian. They're good in Asian dishes but pretty weird in Western-style recipes. Tofu shirataki are white, considerably less chewy, and good in a wide variety of applications. My local health food stores carry them in three widths: fettuccini, spaghetti, and angel hair. I keep the fettuccine and spaghetti widths on hand.

Shirataki come pre-hydrated in a pouch full of liquid. This makes them perfect for our super-quick recipes because you don't have to cook them, only drain and heat them. Snip open the pouch and dump them in a strainer in the sink. You'll notice the liquid smells fishy; you'll want to rinse them. After that, I put them in a microwaveable bowl and give them 90 seconds on high. More liquid will cook out of them, so I drain them againand heat for another 90 seconds, drain yet a third time, and then add whatever sauce I like. This keeps the liquid cooking out of the noodles from diluting the sauce. Shirataki keep up to a year in the fridge, so feel free to stock up.

Glucomannan. This is another finely-milled soluble fiber, similar to xanthan and guar. I've been using it a lot as a thickener this past year and like it a lot. It is available from CarbSmart.com or Amazon.com. Buy it in bulk, not in capsules, and use just like guar or xanthan. Like guar and xanthan, glucomannan will keep pretty much forever, so long as you keep it dry.

15-Minute Eggs

Actually, this is a misnomer—most of these egg dishes will take you well under 15 minutes!

Please, please don't think of eggs as being only for breakfast. Eggs are the ideal low-carb fast food at any time of day. They're cheap, they're tasty, they're nutritious, and they can be prepared in no time flat. With a carton of eggs in the refrigerator, you're never more than a few minutes away from a great meal!

We'll kick things off with omelets, the ultimate low-carb fast food. Once you know how to make an omelet, a whole world of fabulous, quick meals opens up to you.

Dana's Easy Omelet Method

You can learn this quickly. Really you can.

To start, you'll need a good pan. What's a "good pan"? I prefer a medium size skillet with a heavy bottom, sloping sides, and a nonstick surface. However, what I currently have is a 7-inch (18 cm) skillet with a heavy bottom, sloping sides, and a *formerly* nonstick surface. I can still make omelets in it, I just have to use a good shot of nonstick cooking spray. The heavy bottom and sloping sides, however, are essential.

Here's the really important thing to know about making omelets: The word "omelet" comes from a word meaning "to laminate," or to build up layers. And that's exactly what you do—you let a layer of beaten egg cook, and then you lift up the edges and tip the pan so the raw egg runs under the cooked part. You do this all around the edges, of course, so you build it up evenly. The point is, you don't just let the beaten egg lie there in the skillet and wait for it to cook through; the bottom will be hopelessly overdone before the top is set.

So here's the start-to-finish omelet method:

1. First, have your filling ready. If you're using vegetables, you'll want to sauté them first. If you're using cheese, have it grated or sliced and ready to go. If you're making an omelet to use up leftovers (a great idea, by the way), warm them through in the microwave and have them standing by.

2. Spray your omelet pan well with nonstick spray if it doesn't have a good nonstick surface and put it over high heat. While the skillet's heating, grab your eggs (2 is the perfect number for this size pan, but 1 or 3 will work, too) and a bowl, crack the eggs, and beat them with a fork. Don't add any water or milk or anything, just mix them up.

3. Test the heat of the pan. The pan is hot enough when a drop of water thrown in sizzles right away. Add a tablespoon of oil (15 ml) or butter (14 g), slosh it around to cover the bottom, and then pour in the eggs all at once. They should sizzle, too, and immediately start to set. When the bottom layer of egg is set around the edges—this should happen quite quickly—lift the edge using a spatula and tip the pan to let the raw egg flow underneath. Do this all around the edges until there's not enough raw egg to run.

4. Now, turn your burner to the lowest heat if you have a gas stove. (If you have an electric stove, you'll have to have a "warm" burner standing by; electric elements don't cool off fast enough for this job.) Put your filling on one half of the omelet, cover the skillet, and let it sit over very low heat for a minute or two, no more. Peek and see if the raw, shiny egg is gone from the top surface (although you can serve it that way if you like; that's how the French prefer their omelets) and the cheese, if you've used it, is melted. If not, re-cover the skillet and let it sit for another minute or two.

5. When your omelet is done, slip a spatula under the half without the filling and fold it over and then lift the whole thing onto a plate. You could get fancy and tip the pan, letting the filling side of the omelet slide onto the plate and folding the top over as you go, but this takes some practice.

This makes a single-serving omelet. I think it's a lot easier to make several individual omelets than to make one big one, and omelets are so fast to make that it's not that big a deal to make more than one. Anyway, that way you can customize your omelets to each individual's taste. If you're making more than two or three omelets, keep them warm in your oven, set to its very lowest heat, until they're all ready to eat.

Now read on for some ideas for what to put in your omelets!

Omelets

☺ Apple, Bacon, and Blue Cheese Omelet

Here are three of my favorite things—wrapped in eggs, another of my favorite things!

> 3 slices bacon
>
> 1/4 Granny Smith or other crisp, tart apple, thinly sliced
>
> 2 teaspoons butter, divided
>
> 2 eggs, beaten
>
> 1 ounce (28 g) crumbled blue cheese

Start the bacon cooking in the microwave—if you don't own a microwave bacon rack, a glass pie plate will work just fine. (In my microwave, 3 to 4 minutes on High is about right, but microwave power varies.)

While the bacon's cooking, melt 1 teaspoon of butter in your omelet pan over medium-high heat. Add the apples and fry for 2 to 3 minutes per side or until they're slightly golden. Remove the apple slices and keep them on hand.

Melt the remaining butter in the skillet, slosh it about, and make your omelet according to *Dana's Easy Omelet Method* (see page 29), using nonstick cooking spray if necessary. Arrange the fried apples on half the omelet, top with the blue cheese, cover the pan, and turn the burner to low.

Go check on that bacon! If it needs another minute, do that now, while the cheese is melting. Then drain it and crumble it over the now-melted blue cheese. Fold and serve.

Yield: 1 serving, with 6 grams of carbohydrates and 1 gram of fiber, for a total of 5 grams of usable carbs and 23 grams of protein.

☺ Chivey Cheese and Pear Omelets

I never played around with chive cream cheese before working on the new recipes for this book. What a versatile ingredient it is! This omelet is a wonderful, unusual combination of flavors.

1/4 pear

1 tablespoon (14 g) butter

2 eggs

3 tablespoons (38 g) whipped cream cheese with chives

Slice your pear quarter quite thin. Melt the butter in your omelet pan and sauté the pear slices until they've soften a little more. Fork them out onto a plate and reserve.

Scramble up your eggs and pour them into the omelet pan. Cook as described in *Dana's Easy Omelet method.* When the liquid egg has stopped running, turn the burner to low and spoon in the chive cream cheese in little bits, distributing it over half the egg. Top with the pear slices, cover, and cook until the cheese is melted. Fold, plate, and devour!

Yield: 1 serving, with 362 calories, 31 grams fat, 13 grams protein, 9 grams carbohydrate, 1 gram dietary fiber, and 8 grams usable carb.

⊕ Chili Lime Pork Omelet

This is one of those omelets that makes it clear that eggs ain't just for breakfast anymore—this is definitely hearty enough for dinner. The *Chili Lime Pork* is very quick to make and keeps well in a closed container in the fridge.

2 eggs, beaten

1 to 2 teaspoons oil

1/4 batch *Chili Lime Pork Strips* (see page 149)

1/4 avocado, sliced

1/4 cup (29 g) shredded Monterey Jack cheese

Sour cream (optional)

Salsa (optional)

Make your omelet according to *Dana's Easy Omelet Method* (see page 29). Arrange the *Chili Lime Pork* strips on half the omelet and top with the avocado and the cheese. Cover, turn the burner to low, and let it cook for a minute or two to melt the cheese and finish setting the eggs. Fold and serve. Top with sour cream, salsa, or both if desired.

Yield: 1 serving, with 6 grams of carbohydrates and 2 grams of fiber, for a total of 4 grams of usable carbs and 42 grams of protein.

☺ "Clean the Fridge" Omelet

The name is not a joke—I made this omelet up out of whatever I found kicking around in the refrigerator, needing to be used up before it went bad. The results were definitely good enough to make it again.

> 1/2 red bell pepper, cut into thin strips
>
> 1/4 medium onion, thinly sliced
>
> 3 tablespoons (45 ml) olive oil
>
> 2 eggs, beaten
>
> 1 ounce (28 g) jalapeño jack cheese, shredded or sliced
>
> 1/2 avocado, sliced

In your skillet over medium-high heat, sauté the pepper and onion in the oil until the onion is translucent and the pepper is going limp. Remove from the pan and keep on hand. If your pan isn't nonstick, give it a shot of nonstick cooking spray before putting it back on the burner and increasing the heat a touch to high. Make your omelet according to *Dana's Easy Omelet Method* (see page 29). Put the cheese on half the omelet and top with the avocado, then the pepper and onion. Cover, turn the burner to low, and let it cook until the cheese is melted. Fold and serve.

Yield: 1 serving, with 14 grams of carbohydrates and 6 grams of fiber, for a total of 8 grams of usable carbs and 21 grams of protein.

✳ This also contains a whopping 821 milligrams of potassium!

⊕ Cumin Mushroom Omelet

Exotic and wonderful—and even if you're making the *Cumin Mushrooms* from scratch, you'll come in right around the 15-minute mark.

> 2 eggs, beaten
>
> 1 ounce (28 g) Monterey Jack cheese, sliced or shredded
>
> 1/3 batch *Cumin Mushrooms* (see page 265), warmed

Make your omelet according to *Dana's Easy Omelet Method* (see page 29). Put the cheese on half the omelet and then top with the mushrooms. Cover, turn the burner to low, and let it cook for 2 to 3 minutes or until the cheese is melted. Fold and serve.

Yield: 1 serving, with 6 grams of carbohydrates and 1 gram of fiber, for a total of 5 grams of usable carbs and 20 grams of protein.

Variation: A couple of ounces (55 g) of purchased grilled chicken strips make a nice addition to this omelet. If you add the chicken, figure on 1 additional gram of carbohydrate (the chicken strips are marinated before cooking) and 6 additional grams of protein per ounce.

⊕ Caviar and Sour Cream Omelet

Caviar is one of those things—either you like it or you don't. If you do, why not eat it in an omelet? It's sort of an "eggs meet eggs" thing.

> 2 eggs, beaten
>
> 1 tablespoon (16 g) caviar
>
> 3 tablespoons (45 g) sour cream

Make your omelet according to *Dana's Easy Omelet Method* (see page 29). Spread the caviar and sour cream over half the omelet. Cover, turn the burner to low, and cook just another minute or so—you don't want your sour cream to "break." Fold and serve.

Yield: 1 serving, with 4 grams of carbohydrates, no fiber, and 16 grams of protein.

☉ Curried Cheese and Olive Omelets

This was originally a spread for English muffins and the like, but it makes a wicked omelet. I know that this combination of ingredients sounds a little odd, but the flavor is magical.

1 cup (115 g) shredded cheddar cheese

5 or 6 scallions, finely sliced, including the crisp part of the green

I can (4.25 ounces, or 120 g) chopped ripe olives, drained

3 tablespoons (42 g) mayonnaise

1/2 teaspoon curry powder

6 eggs, beaten

Simply plunk the cheese, scallions, olives, mayonnaise, and curry powder in a mixing bowl and combine well. Now, make omelets according to *Dana's Easy Omelet Method* (see page 29), using the cheese-and-olive mixture as the filling. As the 6 eggs suggests, this makes 3 omelets. If there's only one of you, however, just use 2 eggs. The cheese mixture will keep well for a couple of days in a closed container in the refrigerator, letting you make fabulous omelets in far less than 15 minutes for a few days running.

Yield: 3 servings, each with 6 grams of carbohydrates and 3 grams of fiber, for a total of 3 grams of usable carbs and 21 grams of protein.

✳ As a bonus, you get 372 milligrams of calcium!

⊕ Tomato~Mozzarella Omelet

Sliced tomatoes and mozzarella are a time-honored Italian appetizer—and they make a great omelet filling, too.

> 2 eggs, beaten
> 1/3 cup (38 g) shredded mozzarella cheese
> 1/2 small tomato, sliced
> 2 tablespoons (6 g) chopped fresh basil

Make your omelet according to *Dana's Easy Omelet Method* (see page 29). Cover half the omelet with the cheese and then top with the tomato slices. Cover, turn the burner to low, and let it cook for 2 to 3 minutes or until the cheese is melted. Scatter the basil over the filling, fold, and serve.

Yield: 1 serving, with 5 grams of carbohydrates and 1 gram of fiber, for a total of 4 grams of usable carbs and 20 grams of protein.

✯ You'll also get 296 milligrams of potassium and 272 milligrams of calcium.

⊕ Curried Tuna Omelets

These taste really different and really good!

> 2 eggs, beaten
> 1/3 batch *Curried Tuna Salad* (see page 161)

Make your omelet according to *Dana's Easy Omelet Method* (see page 29). Cover half the omelet with the tuna salad. Cover, turn the burner to low, and cook long enough to warm through. Fold and serve.

Yield: 1 serving, with 7 grams of carbohydrates and 2 grams of fiber, for a total of 5 grams of usable carbs and 33 grams of protein.

⊕ Kasseri Tapenade Omelet

This is full of cool Greek flavors! Look for jars of tapenade, an olive relish, in big grocery stores. Kasseri is a Greek cheese; all my local grocery stores carry it, so I'm guessing yours do, too.

> 2 to 3 teaspoons (10 to 15 ml) olive oil
>
> 2 eggs, beaten
>
> 1 ounce (28 g) kasseri cheese, sliced or shredded
>
> 1 1/2 tablespoons (12 g) tapenade

Make your omelet according to *Dana's Easy Omelet Method* (see page 29). Cover half the omelet with the cheese and then top with the tapenade. Cover, turn the burner to low, and let it cook for a couple of minutes until the cheese is melted. Fold and serve.

Yield: 1 serving, with 4 grams of carbohydrates, no fiber, and 18 grams of protein.

☉ Unborn Buffalo Wings

I had leftover buffalo wing sauce and thought of this. It turned out great! You could use bottled buffalo wing sauce if you have some on hand, but half-and-half of butter and Louisiana-style hot sauce is the canonical recipe.

> 1/2 tablespoon bacon grease
>
> 2 eggs
>
> 3 tablespoons (24 g) crumbled blue cheese
>
> 1 tablespoon (15 ml) Louisiana-style hot sauce
>
> 1 tablespoon (14 g) butter

Make your omelet according to *Dana's Easy Omelet Method* (see page 29) using the bacon grease for the fat. Fill with the blue cheese.

While your omelet is covered on low heat, melting the cheese, melt the butter with the Tabasco sauce in a small saucepan or nuke for a minute in a custard cup. Stir them together well.

When your omelet's done, fold and plate, and then top with the sauce and eat. YUMMY!

Yield: 1 serving, with 384 calories, 34 grams fat, 17 grams protein, 2 grams carbohydrate, 0 grams dietary fiber, and 2 grams usable carb.

Scrambles

Think of scrambles as omelets for the faint of heart. And please, feel free to experiment with scrambles of your own! The variety of things that taste good when added to scrambled eggs is never-ending.

⊕ Smoked Salmon and Goat Cheese Scramble

Sounds fancy, I know, but this takes almost no time and is very impressive. It's terrific to make for a special brunch or a late-night supper. A simple green salad with a classic vinaigrette dressing would be perfect with this.

> 4 eggs
> 1/2 cup (120 ml) heavy cream
> 1 teaspoon dried dill weed
> 4 scallions
> 1/4 pound (115 g) chevre (goat cheese)
> 1/4 pound (115 g) moist smoked salmon
> 1 to 2 tablespoons (14 to 28 g) butter

Whisk the eggs together with the cream and dill weed. Slice the scallions thin, including the crisp part of the green. Cut the chevre—it will have a texture similar to cream cheese—into little hunks. Coarsely crumble the smoked salmon.

In a big (preferably nonstick) skillet, melt the butter over medium-high heat. (If your skillet doesn't have a nonstick surface, give it a shot of nonstick cooking spray before adding the butter.) When the butter's melted, add the scallions first and sauté them for just a minute. Add the eggs and cook, stirring frequently, until they're halfway set—about 1 minute to 90 seconds. Add the chevre and smoked salmon, continue cooking and stirring until the eggs are set, and serve.

Yield: 3 servings, each with 5 grams of carbohydrates and 1 gram of fiber, for a total of 4 grams of usable carbs and 27 grams of protein.

☉ Deviled Ham and Eggs

If you don't have leftover ham lying around the house, you can buy modest-size chunks of pre-cooked ham in any grocery store. It's useful stuff!

1/2 tablespoon butter

1/2 cup (75 g) smallish ham cubes

1/4 cup (40 g) chopped onion

3 eggs

1 teaspoon spicy brown or Dijon mustard

1 teaspoon prepared horseradish

Melt the butter in a small skillet over medium heat. Add the ham and onion and sauté until the onion is translucent and the ham has a touch of gold. Scramble the eggs with the mustard and horseradish and pour them over the ham and onion in the skillet. Scramble until the eggs are set and serve.

Yield: 1 serving, with 8 grams of carbohydrates (less if you use really low-carb ham) and 1 gram of fiber, for a total of 7 grams of usable carbs and 29 grams of protein.

⊕ Parmesan Rosemary Eggs

This is so simple and so wonderful. If you like Italian food, you have to try this. It's also easy to double or triple.

> 3 eggs
>
> 2 tablespoons (28 ml) heavy cream
>
> 1/4 cup (25 g) grated Parmesan cheese
>
> 1/2 teaspoon ground rosemary*
>
> 1/2 teaspoon minced garlic
>
> 1/2 tablespoon butter

* You can use whole, dried rosemary, but you'll have little needles in your food. If you do use whole rosemary, increase the amount to 1 teaspoon.

Whisk together the eggs, cream, cheese, rosemary, and garlic. Put a medium-size skillet over medium-high heat (if it isn't nonstick, give it a shot of nonstick cooking spray first). When the pan is hot, add the butter, give the egg mixture one last stir to make sure the cheese hasn't settled to the bottom, and then pour the egg mixture into the skillet. Scramble until the eggs are set and serve.

Yield: 1 serving, with 3 grams of carbohydrates, a trace of fiber, and 25 grams of protein.

⊕ Blue Eggs

Wow—here's some scrambled eggs with blue cheese and herbs. Yum!

> 4 eggs
>
> 2 tablespoons (16 g) crumbled blue cheese
>
> 3 scallions, finely sliced
>
> 2 tablespoons (8 g) chopped fresh parsley
>
> 1/8 teaspoon dried marjoram
>
> 1/8 teaspoon dried thyme

Just scramble up the eggs, add the cheese, scallions, parsley, marjoram, and thyme, and stir it all up. Give your big, heavy skillet a shot of nonstick cooking spray, heat it over medium-high heat, and pour in the egg and cheese mixture. Scramble until set and serve.

Yield: 1 or 2 servings. Assuming 2 servings, each will have 3 grams of carbohydrates and 1 gram of fiber, for a total of 2 grams of usable carbs and 13 grams of protein.

⊕Moroccan Scramble

With all these vegetables, this is a meal in itself. It's exotic and fabulous.

> 1 tablespoon (15 ml) olive oil
>
> 1/4 cup (40 g) chopped onion
>
> 1/2 teaspoon minced garlic or 1 clove garlic, crushed
>
> 1 tablespoon (8 g) tapenade
>
> 1/4 cup (45 g) canned diced tomatoes
>
> 3 eggs
>
> 1/2 teaspoon ground cumin
>
> 2 tablespoons (2 g) chopped fresh cilantro
>
> Salt and pepper

In a skillet, heat the olive oil over high heat and start sautéing the onion and garlic. When the onion is translucent, add the tapenade and tomatoes and stir. Now, whisk the eggs with the cumin and pour the eggs into the vegetable mixture. Scramble until mostly set and then add the cilantro and scramble until done. Salt and pepper to taste and serve.

Yield: 1 serving, with 11 grams of carbohydrates and 1 gram of fiber, for a total of 10 grams of usable carbs and 18 grams of protein.

⊕ French Country Scramble

This is for anyone who doesn't think that eggs can be elegant.

> 4 ounces (115 g) sliced mushrooms
>
> 3 scallions, coarsely sliced
>
> 1 tablespoon (14 g) butter
>
> 2 canned artichoke hearts, chopped
>
> 6 eggs
>
> 1/2 cup (60 g) shredded Gruyère cheese

If you haven't purchased your mushrooms already sliced, slice then up while you slice the scallions. In a large, heavy skillet over medium-high heat, sauté the mushrooms and scallions in the butter. When the mushrooms have turned darker, add the artichoke hearts (I just slice mine right into the skillet) and stir the whole thing up. Then beat the eggs, add them to the skillet, and scramble the whole thing. When the eggs are about half-set, add the cheese and scramble until done. Serve.

Yield: 2 or 3 servings. Assuming 3 servings, each will have 10 grams of carbohydrates and 4 grams of fiber, for a total of 6 grams of usable carbs and 19 grams of protein. Note: Keep in mind that much of the carbohydrate in artichokes is in the form of inulin, about the lowest-impact carbohydrate yet discovered, so the blood sugar impact is less than the numbers would imply—which is pretty low to begin with.

☉ Huevos Con El Sabor de Chiles Rellenos

Chiles Rellenos—green chilies stuffed with cheese, dipped in batter, and then fried—are irresistible and very time-consuming to make. However, since the traditional batter is egg-rich, it occurred to me to incorporate the chilies and the cheese into a scramble. It's delicious! If you haven't tried canned green chilies, you should know that they're only slightly spicy—this recipe won't leave you gasping and reaching for a glass of water.

6 eggs

1/4 cup (30 g) canned diced green chilies

1 tablespoon (14 g) butter or oil (15 ml)

4 ounces (115 g) Monterey Jack cheese, cut into small chunks

Beat the eggs with the chilies. Spray a large, heavy skillet with nonstick cooking spray and put it over medium-high heat. When the skillet is hot, add the butter or oil and slosh it around to coat the bottom of the skillet.

Pour in the beaten eggs with chilies and scramble them until they're about half-set. Add the chunks of Monterey Jack cheese, continue scrambling until set, and then serve.

Yield: 2 or 3 servings. Assuming 2 servings, each will have 4 grams of carbohydrates, a trace of fiber, and 31 grams of protein.

☺Hangtown Fry

This is a very famous dish originating, I believe, in the Gold Rush days of California.

  8 large oysters

  2 tablespoons (16 g) low-carb bake mix or 2 tablespoons (20 g)
     rice protein powder

  4 tablespoons (55 g) butter

  4 eggs

  2 tablespoons (28 ml) cream

  2 tablespoons (10 g) grated Parmesan cheese

  2 tablespoons (8 g) chopped fresh parsley

Coat the oysters with the bake mix or protein powder, either by putting the bake mix or protein powder in a shallow dish and rolling the oysters in it or by shaking them in a small brown paper bag with the mix in it.

Melt the butter over medium heat in a large, heavy skillet. Add the oysters and fry until golden all over, about 5 to 7 minutes.

While the oysters are frying, beat the eggs and the cream together. When the oysters are golden, pour the beaten eggs into the skillet and scramble until set. Divide between 2 serving plates, sprinkle a tablespoon (5 g) of Parmesan and a tablespoon (4 g) of parsley over each portion, and serve.

Yield: 2 servings, each with 5 grams of carbohydrates and 1 gram of fiber, for a total of 4 grams of usable carbs and 21 grams of protein.

⊕ Cottage Egg Scramble

Eggs scrambled with cottage cheese are surprisingly good, and of course the cottage cheese adds nutrients the eggs lack—most notably calcium. With a salad on the side, this is a great simple supper for a tired night.

    4 eggs
    1/2 cup (115 g) small-curd cottage cheese
    1/8 teaspoon dried basil
    1/2 green pepper, finely chopped
    1 tablespoon butter
    1/4 cup (29 g) shredded cheddar cheese

Beat the eggs and cottage cheese together and stir in the basil. In a large, heavy skillet over medium-high heat, sauté the green pepper in the butter (you might want to give that skillet a shot of nonstick cooking spray first). When the pepper is getting a little soft, add the egg mixture and scramble. When the eggs are almost set, add the cheddar and continue scrambling until the eggs are completely set. Serve.

Yield: 2 servings, each with 5 grams of carbohydrates and 1 gram of fiber, for a total of 4 grams of usable carbs and 23 grams of protein.

☉ Chipotle Eggs

Smoky and complex, chipotle peppers—smoked jalapeños—are very special, and they make these eggs very special, too. Personally, I think a side of avocado slices with a little lime or lemon juice would be nice with this.

1/2 cup (80 g) finely chopped onion

1/2 teaspoon minced garlic or 1 clove garlic, crushed

1 tablespoon (15 ml) oil

2 small chipotle peppers canned in adobo sauce, finely minced—about 2 teaspoons

6 eggs

1/2 cup (58 g) shredded Monterey Jack cheese

Spray a large, heavy skillet with nonstick cooking spray, place it over medium-high heat, and start sautéing the onion and garlic in the oil. When the onion is translucent, add the chopped chipotles, stir them in, and let the whole thing cook for another minute. (This is a good time to break and scramble the eggs.)

Pour the eggs into the skillet and scramble until nearly set. Scatter the cheese evenly over the top, turn the burner to low, cover the skillet, and let it keep cooking until the cheese is melted—just a minute or two. Serve.

Yield: 2 or 3 servings. Assuming 2 servings, each will have 5 grams of carbohydrates and 1 gram of fiber, for a total of 4 grams of usable carbs and 24 grams of protein.

✳ This also contains 285 milligrams of calcium and 248 milligrams of potassium. (There's even more potassium if you have those avocado slices!)

⊕ Houbyfest Eggs

"What the heck is 'Houbyfest'?" I hear you cry. "Houby" is Czech for "mushroom," and Houbyfest is an annual mushroom celebration in the heavily Bohemian Chicago suburb of Berwyn. This dish is so loaded with mushrooms—as much mushroom as egg—that the name seemed appropriate.

    8 ounces (225 g) sliced mushrooms

    2 tablespoons (28 g) butter

    1 teaspoon dried thyme

    1/2 teaspoon minced garlic or 1 clove garlic, crushed

    2 scallions, sliced

    6 eggs

    2 tablespoons (8 g) chopped fresh parsley (optional)

In a large, heavy skillet, sauté the mushrooms in the butter over medium-high heat. When the mushrooms have turned dark, stir in the thyme, garlic, and scallions and let them cook for a minute or two while you crack and scramble the eggs. Then pour the eggs into the skillet, scramble, and serve.
A little fresh parsley scattered over this is nice but not essential.

Yield: 2 or 3 servings. Assuming 2 servings, each will have 9 grams of carbohydrates and 2 grams of fiber, for a total of 7 grams of usable carbs and 19 grams of protein.

☆ This dish has 633 milligrams potassium!

⊕ Insta-Quiche

As the name implies, this has a similar flavor to a classic Quiche Lorraine, but it cooks entirely within our 15 minute limit.

    8 slices bacon

    5 eggs

    1/2 cup (120 ml) half and half

    1/2 teaspoon salt

    1/4 teaspoon pepper

1 pinch ground nutmeg

1 tablespoon (28 ml) dry vermouth

1 tablespoon (14 g) butter

8 ounces (225 g) shredded Swiss cheese

Place a 10 inch (25 cm) nonstick skillet over medium heat. Let it heat.

Lay the bacon on a microwave bacon rack or in a Pyrex baking dish that fits in your microwave. Stick in it the microwave on high for 8 to 9 minutes. (The length of time will depend a bit on your microwave.)

In a medium mixing bowl, whisk together the eggs, half and half, salt, pepper, nutmeg, and vermouth.

Plunk your butter in your now-hot skillet and slosh it around as it melts, to coat the bottom. Now pour in your egg mixture. Use a spatula—preferably one for nonstick skillets—to gently stir the eggs around, pulling back the part that's setting and letting the liquid egg run underneath. It won't work like an omelet, where it sets up firm enough that you can lift the whole edge. Just scramble them gently until they're about half-set, half-liquid.

Spread the eggs out evenly in the skillet and sprinkle the shredded cheese over the top. Cover the skillet and turn the burner to low. (If you have an electric stove, you'll need to shift your pan to a low burner.) Turn on the broiler and set the rack four inches below it.

When the bacon is done, take it out, put it on a paper towel to drain if you used the Pyrex pan, and let it cool just a minute or two. Then crumble it, or easier, you can use your kitchen shears to snip it into bits. Uncover your Insta-Quiche and sprinkle the bacon bits evenly over the top.

Now slide the whole thing under the broiler for just a minute until you're sure the top is set and then cut in wedges and serve.

Yield: 4 servings, each with 438 calories, 34 grams fat (70.3% calories from fat), 28 grams protein, 4 grams carbohydrate, trace dietary fiber, 315 mg cholesterol, and 727 mg sodium.

Note: This requires some coordination and came in just at the fifteen minute mark. But even if you take sixteen minutes, it's worth it.

⊕ Eggs Fu Yong

This can be made on the stove top, is quick and cheap to make, uses up any sort of leftover meat, is high in protein and low in carbohydrates, needs no side dishes, is infinitely variable, and tastes good to boot! How much more can you ask from a recipe? Because this recipe can be varied so much, what I've given you is more a guideline than hard and fast rules.

    4 eggs
    2 teaspoons dry sherry
    1 tablespoon (15 ml) soy sauce
    Peanut oil, or other bland oil for frying
    1/2 teaspoon grated gingerroot
    2 to 3 ounces (55 to 85 g) leftover cooked meat, cut into small strips* or 2 to
        3 ounces (55 to 85 g) canned chunk turkey, chicken, or ham, or canned
        shrimp, or crabmeat
    1 cup (70 g) Napa cabbage or (90 g) green cabbage, finely shredded, or bagged
        coleslaw mix (90 g), or 1 cup (104 g) bean sprouts, or some combination of
        the two
    1/4 cup (18 g) mushrooms, canned or fresh, finely chopped
    1/4 cup (40 g) onion or (25 g) scallions, finely minced
    1/4 cup (33 g) bamboo shoots, cut into matchstick strips

* Use ham, pork, turkey, chicken, or shrimp—whatever you've got. If they're little bitty shrimp, leave 'em whole. If they're great big shrimp, chop them coarsely.

Beat the eggs with the sherry and the soy sauce. Set aside. In a large skillet, heat a few tablespoons (28 to 45 ml) of oil over high heat. Add the ginger, then the meat and vegetables. Stir-fry until the onion is translucent and the cabbage or bean sprouts are tender-crisp. Stir the meat and vegetables into the seasoned eggs. Add another few tablespoons (28 to 45 ml) of oil to the skillet and heat.

Ladle in about 1/2 cup (120 ml) of the egg mixture at a time and fry on both sides until the egg is set.

You can cook this in a wok if you want to be terribly authentic, but I actually find that a skillet is a lot easier for this recipe.

Yield: 2 servings. The carb count will vary a little, but each serving will have close to 6 grams of carbohydrates and 2 grams of fiber, for a total of 4 grams of usable carbs and 26 grams of protein.

Fried Eggs

⊕ Asparagi All'Uovo

This Italian dish turns a couple of eggs into a light supper. This looks like a lot of instructions, but none of the steps takes much time.

> 1 pound (455 g) asparagus
> 1/4 cup (60 ml) olive oil
> 1/2 teaspoon minced garlic or 1 clove garlic, crushed
> 1/2 cup (50 g) grated Parmesan cheese
> 8 eggs

Start by snapping the bottoms off the asparagus where they break naturally. Put the asparagus in a microwaveable casserole or a glass pie plate. Add a couple of tablespoons of water and cover. (Use plastic wrap or a plate to cover a pie plate.) Microwave on High for 3 to 4 minutes.

While the asparagus is cooking, stir the garlic into the olive oil.

When the asparagus is done, drain it. If you have 4 single-serving oven-proof dishes long enough to hold asparagus, they're ideal for this recipe—divide the asparagus between the 4 dishes. If not, you'll need to use a rectangular glass baking dish. Arrange the asparagus in 4 groups in the baking dish.

Whether you're using the individual dishes or the single baking dish, drizzle each serving of asparagus with the garlic and olive oil. Salt and pepper lightly and divide the cheese between the 4 servings. Put the asparagus under the broiler, about 4 inches (10 cm) from low heat. Let it broil for 4 to 5 minutes.

While the asparagus is broiling, fry the eggs to your liking. Either use your biggest skillet to do them all at once or divide them between two skillets.

When the Parmesan is lightly golden, take the asparagus out of the broiler. If you've cooked it in one baking dish, use a big spatula to carefully transfer each serving of asparagus to a plate. Top each serving of asparagus with 2 fried eggs and serve.

Yield: 4 servings, each with 4 grams of carbohydrates and 1 gram of fiber, for a total of 3 grams of usable carbs and 16 grams of protein. If you'd like 22 grams of protein, add a third egg to each serving.

⊕ Colorful Eggs on a Plate

I wanted to come up with something completely microwaved, though I can't really explain why. This is quite good, and heaven knows it's quick.

> 1/4 red bell pepper
>
> 1/4 green bell pepper
>
> 1/4 onion
>
> 3 ounces (85 g) ham
>
> 1 tablespoon (15 g) bacon grease or melted butter
>
> 2 eggs
>
> 3 tablespoons (22 g) shredded Monterey Jack cheese

Cut the veggies and ham into a few chunks, throw them in the food processor, and pulse until chopped to a medium consistency.

Spray a microwaveable plate with a rim with nonstick cooking spray and dump the veggie-ham mixture on it. Drizzle the bacon grease or butter over it, stir it all around, and then spread it in an even layer. Nuke on high for 1 minute.

While that's happening, scramble up your eggs in a small bowl. When the microwave beeps, pour the eggs over the veggies and ham. Put it back in and nuke for another 2 to 3 minutes or until the eggs are mostly set.

Sprinkle the cheese over the top and nuke again for another 1 to 2 minutes or until the cheese is melted and then eat.

Yield: 1 serving, with 510 calories, 37 grams fat, 32 grams protein, 10 grams carbohydrate, 2 grams dietary fiber, and 8 grams usable carb.

⊕ Ham and Eggs with Veg

The recipe I adapted this from—from a 1960s cookbook—swore this was a Spanish recipe. I don't know if it's anything vaguely resembling Spanish cooking, but it's tasty, quick, filling, and unusual.

> 1/2 cup (75 g) frozen peas
>
> 1/2 medium onion, diced
>
> 3 medium fresh mushrooms, chopped
>
> 4 tablespoons (60 ml) olive oil, divided
>
> 3/4 cup ham, cut into 1/2-inch (1.3 cm) cubes
>
> 4 eggs
>
> 4 green olives

Put the peas in a microwaveable bowl, add just little water, cover with a saucer, and nuke on high for four minutes.

In the meantime, dice your onion, chop your mushrooms, and start them sautéing in a medium-sized skillet over medium heat using 2 tablespoons (28 ml) of the olive oil.

While all that is cooking, cube your ham. Throw it in with the onions and mushrooms and stir it all up. Let it sauté a bit longer.

Fry the eggs in the rest of the olive oil in another pan. You want the whites set but the yolks still runny.

By now the microwave has beeped! Stir the peas into the ham and veg mixture and let them cook with it a touch longer.

Pit and chop the olives.

Okay, divide the ham mixture onto two plates and top each with two fried eggs. Scatter some chopped olive over each portion and serve.

Yield: 2 servings, each with 517 calories, 42 grams fat, 23 grams protein, 12 grams carbohydrate, 3 grams dietary fiber, and 9 grams usable carb.

Something Different

⊕ Blintzlets

This falls somewhere between a blintz and an omelet—hence the name.
These are not dirt-low in carbs, but they're really yummy. They can be a
special breakfast—you'll want to add a little more protein on the side,
maybe some ham—or even a light dessert.

> 1 cup (225 g) cottage cheese*
>
> 2 tablespoons (30 g) sour cream
>
> 1/2 teaspoon vanilla extract
>
> 1 tablespoon (1.5 g) Splenda
>
> 4 eggs
>
> 1/4 cup (40 g) vanilla whey protein powder
>
> 6 tablespoons (120 g) low-sugar strawberry preserves

* I use 4% fat cottage cheese; don't drop below 2%.

Put the cottage cheese, sour cream, vanilla, and Splenda in your food processor with
the S-blade in place. Process until smooth.

Put the eggs and the protein powder in a blender and whirl for 20 seconds or so.

Heat an 8- or 9-inch (20 or 23 cm) nonstick skillet over medium-high heat. Make
sure it's hot before you cook! Even though it's nonstick, spray it with nonstick cooking spray. Now, pour in a small puddle of the egg mixture and swirl the pan to coat
the whole bottom—the idea is to use just enough of the egg mixture to cover the
bottom of the skillet with a thin but solid layer. Cook until the top of the egg is
set—this takes only a minute or so—then turn briefly. The protein powder makes
this mixture very fragile, so be careful.

Lay the thin, eggy pancake on a plate, spread 1 tablespoon (20 g) of the preserves on
one half and spoon 3 tablespoons (42 g) of the cottage cheese mixture over it. Fold
and serve. Repeat.

Yield: Makes 6, each with 9 grams of carbohydrates and 11 grams of protein. You
can cut the carb count of each serving 3 grams by using just 1/2 tablespoon of
preserves in each one. Or you could thaw 1/2 cup (128 g) of frozen unsweetened

strawberries, mash them with a tablespoon or two (1.5 to 3 g) of Splenda, and use them in place of the preserves. This would save 5 grams of carbs per serving—but you'll be pushing that 15-minute time limit.

⏲ Egg and Cheese Pancakes

I admit it, getting all of these done with the 15 minute deadline will take a big griddle. But you can easily have the first round done in a big skillet finished within that time.

> 1 cup (225 g) creamed cottage cheese
>
> 4 eggs
>
> 1 teaspoon baking powder
>
> 1 teaspoon vanilla
>
> 1/4 teaspoon salt
>
> 1/4 cup (31 g) coconut flour
>
> 1 tablespoon (1.5 g) Splenda, or liquid sucralose to equal 1 tablespoon in
>   sweetness

First, put the biggest darned skillet or griddle you can find on to heat over medium-high burners. (If it can span two burners, so much the better!)

Now simply assemble everything else in your blender and run until you have a smooth, thick batter.

Cook as you would any pancake, turning when the edges look dry and the bubbles that pop leave holes. Serve with butter and low sugar jelly or mixed Splenda granular or erythriltol and cinnamon.

Yield: Makes 15 pancakes, each with 50 calories, 2 grams fat, 4 grams protein, 4 grams carbohydrate, 2 grams dietary fiber, and 2 grams usable carb.

⏰ Chipotle-Bacon Breakfast Burrito

This dish is super-tasty and filling enough to be a quick supper. A little fresh cilantro would be nice here, too, but it's hardly essential.

> 2 slices bacon
>
> 1 tablespoon (10 g) diced onion
>
> 1 chipotle chile canned in adobo
>
> 1 tablespoon (15 g) bacon grease
>
> 1 low carb tortilla, 6-inch (15 cm) size
>
> 3 eggs
>
> 2 tablespoons (30 g) sour cream
>
> 1/4 cup (29 g) shredded Monterey Jack cheese

Lay your bacon on a microwave bacon rack or in a Pyrex pie plate and nuke it on high for two to three minutes.

In the meantime, dice your onion and chop up your chipotle. Start sautéing them in the bacon grease over medium heat.

When the bacon is crisp, pull it out and drain it. Lay your tortilla on a microwaveable plate and scatter the cheese evenly over it. Nuke for 1 minute—70% power is right in my microwave; you're just melting the cheese.

In the meantime, break your eggs, scramble them, and pour them over the onion and chipotle. Stir until set.

Okay, it's time to assemble your burrito: Pull your tortilla with the melted cheese out of the microwave. Arrange the scrambled eggs down the middle, top with a teaspoon or two of the adobo sauce from the chilies, and then dot with the sour cream. Top with the cooked bacon, wrap, and devour!

Yield: 1 serving, with 610 calories, 49 grams fat, 34 grams protein, 15 grams carbohydrate, 9 grams dietary fiber, and 6 grams usable carb.

⊕ Vedgeree

Kedgeree is a traditional dish made with rice; flaked, smoked mackerel or halibut; and hard-boiled eggs. I wanted to decarb it, but smoked mackerel and halibut are hard to come by, and I refuse to include impossible-to-find ingredients. Then I found a recipe for "Vedgeree," a vegetarian take-off, so I decarbed it, and it was yummy. This recipe will make a satisfying one-dish meal out of a couple of hard-boiled eggs. You do keep hard-boiled eggs in the fridge, don't you?

> 1/4 head cauliflower
>
> 1/2 cup (25 g) frozen cross-cut green beans
>
> 1/4 cup (40 g) chopped onion
>
> 1 cup (70 g) sliced mushrooms
>
> 1/2 tablespoon butter
>
> 2 hard-boiled eggs
>
> Salt and pepper

Run the cauliflower through the shredding blade of a food processor. Put the cauliflower in a microwaveable dish, put the frozen green beans on top, add a couple of tablespoons (28 ml) of water, cover, and microwave on High for 7 minutes.

While the cauliflower and beans are cooking, sauté the onion and mushrooms in the butter until the onions are limp and translucent and the mushrooms have turned dark. Peel the eggs, quarter them lengthwise, and set them aside.

When the cauliflower and beans are done, pull them out, drain them, and stir them into the mushrooms and onions. Salt and pepper to taste. Place the hard-boiled egg quarters on top of the vegetables, turn the burner to low, cover the pan, and let the whole thing cook for just another minute or two to heat the eggs through. Serve.

Yield: 1 serving, with 14 grams of carbohydrates and 4 grams of fiber, for a total of 10 grams of usable carbs and 16 grams of protein.

☺Microwave-Baked Eggs with Mushrooms

Finally! I microwave-baked eggs and they came out right! They were super-tasty, in fact. Don't worry about the teeny bit of wiggly-ness in the whites when these come out of the microwave; it'll cook as you stir the egg in with the mushrooms.

> 5 mushrooms
>
> 1/4 onion
>
> 2 tablespoons (28 g) plus 1 teaspoon (5 g) butter
>
> 2 eggs

Throw the mushrooms and onion in your food processor and pulse to chop medium-fine. Scrape this mixture into a microwaveable bowl, add the 2 tablespoons (28 g) of butter cut into bits, cover, and nuke on high for a minute.

Spoon the mushroom mixture into two ramekins, about 3 inches (7.5 cm) across and 2 inches (5 cm) deep—big custard cups will do, too. Break an egg into each one and use a sharp knife point to just barely pierce the yolk on each one. Salt and pepper and dot with the remaining butter.

Cover the two dishes loosely with paper toweling, nuke on high for 2 minutes, and then serve. (The time may be a little different depending on the power of your microwave. My whites were mostly set, my yolks still soft.)

Yield: 2 servings, each with 201 calories, 18 grams fat, 7 grams protein, 4 grams carbohydrate, 1 gram dietary fiber, and 3 grams usable carb.

15~Minute Tortilla Tricks

Yes, there are low-carbohydrate tortillas! They're made by La Tortilla Factory, and they're loaded with fiber, which is why they're low carb—each tortilla has 12 grams of carbohydrate and 9 grams of fiber, for a total of just 3 grams of usable carbs.

As the popularity of low-carb dieting has increased, these low-carb tortillas have become easier to find in stores—I know a couple of places that carry them here in Bloomington, Indiana, and it's not like we're the retail capital of the universe. Look around. If you can't find them, consider asking a local health food store to special order them for you—most health food stores are really helpful about special orders, and if enough people ask for the tortillas, the store may start carrying them as a matter of course.

If even that fails, go online and do a search for "low-carbohydrate tortillas." You'll find plenty of e-tailers happy to ship them to you.

Low-carb tortillas are not exactly like either flour or corn tortillas; they have a flavor and texture of their own. We really enjoy them, and they sure are versatile! With a package of low-carb tortillas in the house and some cheese in the fridge, you've got a quick meal, any time.

I have tried making low-carb tortilla chips by cutting low-carb tortillas into wedges and frying them. The results were edible, but not great—tough, and a bit cardboardy. Feel free to try it if you'd like. Me, I'd rather have nuts or fiber crackers or something.

Since I didn't like the low-carb tortilla chips, I haven't tried frying these low-carb tortillas to make taco shells or tostadas. I think the low-carb tortillas are best left in their original soft-and-pliable state. This chapter will teach you a few ways to use them.

⊕ Quesadillas

Is there anyone left who hasn't tried this Mexican version of the grilled cheese sandwich? If you'd like to make a single-serving quesadilla, use a single tortilla, cover half of it with cheese, and fold it over. Heck, you can use this method for all your quesadillas if you like; I just find the sandwiching method easier.

>   2 low-carb tortillas
>
>   4 ounces (115 g) cheese, sliced or shredded

* Mexican Queso Quesadilla is the classic choice, but Monterey Jack, jalapeño jack, and cheddar are all great, too.

Put one tortilla in the bottom of a large, heavy, dry skillet over medium heat. Spread the cheese over it, and place the other tortilla on top. Let it cook a few minutes until the cheese is starting to melt. Carefully flip the whole thing and let it cook on the other side until the cheese is well-melted. Remove from the skillet, cut the quesadilla into quarters—a pizza cutter works well—and serve.

Yield: 2 servings, each with 12 grams of carbohydrates and 9 grams of fiber, for a total of 3 grams of usable carbs and 19 grams of protein.

✫ Each serving also contains 463 milligrams of calcium!

Quesadillas Picantes

I love jalapeños, so this recipe is one of my personal favorites.

Make your quesadilla as described, but place slices of canned jalapeño on top of the cheese and let them melt into the cheese.

Yield: 2 servings, each with 13 grams of carbohydrates and 9 grams of fiber, for a total of 4 grams of usable carbs and 19 grams of protein.

☺ Mondo Giganto Quesadilla-from-Hell

Zowie—this is a serious meal. Thank my husband for the name—he took one look at this big, thick quesadilla, and that's what he called it.

2 low-carb tortillas

3 ounces (85 g) shredded Monterey Jack cheese

3 ounces (85 g) purchased grilled chicken strips

1/2 tablespoon canned sliced jalapeños

1/4 ripe avocado, sliced

Place one of the tortillas in a large, heavy, dry skillet. Spread half the shredded cheese on it, then top with the chicken, jalapeños, and avocado slices, and top with the rest of the cheese. Place the second tortilla on top. Toast over medium heat, with a tilted lid, for 3 to 4 minutes, or until the cheese is melting. Flip your Quesadilla-from-Hell carefully—a few bits may escape from the sides because it's so full of yumminess; just tuck the bits back in. Continue toasting until all the cheese is melted. I find it easiest to use a pizza cutter to cut this in quarters right in the pan (turn the heat off first). The quarters are far easier to transfer to plates than the whole bursting-at-the-seams thing.

Yield: 2 servings, each with 14 grams of carbohydrates and 10 grams of fiber, for a total of 4 grams of usable carbs and 29 grams of protein.

Tip: If you don't have purchased grilled chicken strips in the house, you can, of course, just throw a boneless, skinless chicken breast in your electric tabletop grill for 5 to 6 minutes and then slice it up. This is good without the chicken, too, although lower in protein, of course. (The carb count drops 1 gram for each ounce of chicken.)

⊕ Gorgonzola and Pecan Quesadillas

This makes a casually elegant snack or starter for company, but it's too good not to make it just for yourself.

 1/4 cup (28 g) chopped pecans

 2 teaspoons butter, divided

 1/2 teaspoon Cajun seasoning

 3 ounces (85 g) crumbled gorgonzola cheese

 2 low carb tortillas, large

Over medium-low heat, sauté the pecans in the butter, stirring often, until they smell toasty. Stir in the Cajun seasoning and remove from the heat before they can scorch!

In a big skillet over medium heat, lay one tortilla flat, spread the crumbled gorgonzola evenly over it, and then layer in the pecans. Top with the second tortilla. Let it cook 4 to 5 minutes and then flip carefully. Give it another 3 to 4 minutes. Cut into quarters to remove from the skillet.

Yield: 2 servings, each with 367 calories, 29 grams fat, 10 grams protein, 24 grams carbohydrate, 17 grams dietary fiber, and 7 grams usable carb.

⊕ Vermont Quesadillas

If you've ever been to Vermont, you know that every store you pass, no matter how small, has a sign advertising two things: Vermont cheddar and maple syrup. I found myself wondering how I could combine these into a single dish and came up with this—though, of course, Vermonters would consider the sugar-free pancake syrup heresy. It's an unusual and wonderful combination. If you can't get Vermont cheddar, use the best and sharpest cheddar you can get, preferably undyed.

> 1/4 cup (30 g) chopped walnuts
>
> 2 low carb tortillas, large
>
> 3 ounces (85 g) extra sharp Vermont cheddar cheese
>
> 1 tablespoon (20 g) sugar-free pancake syrup
>
> 1/4 teaspoon hot sauce or to taste

Lay your chopped walnuts on a microwaveable plate and give them 90 seconds or so on high.

In the meantime, put your big skillet over medium heat and lay one of the tortillas over it. Using a box grater, shred the cheese right onto the tortilla.

By now the walnuts are toasted. Pull them out of the microwave and sprinkle them evenly over the cheese. Top with the second tortilla and let the whole thing cook a couple of minutes.

Flip carefully and continue cooking until the cheese is melted and the tortilla has a few browned spots.

In the meantime, mix the pancake syrup with the hot sauce. Divide into two small dishes.

When the quesadilla's done, cut it in quarters right there in the skillet and put the quarters on two plates along with the pancake syrup mixture. To eat, dip the edge of the quesadilla in just a teeny bit of the pancake syrup before each bite.

Yield: 2 servings, each with 350 calories, 26 grams fat, 14 grams protein, 22 grams carbohydrate, 15 grams dietary fiber, and 7 grams usable carb.

⏱ Tortilla Pizza

This makes a great snack or light lunch. Keep in mind that the sauce is the highest carb part of this; don't go increasing the quantity.

> 1 low-carb tortilla
>
> 1 1/2 tablespoons (23 g) no-sugar-added pizza sauce
>
> 1/2 cup (60 g) shredded mozzarella cheese

Place the tortilla on the baking tray of the toaster oven. Spread the pizza sauce over it and then top with the cheese. Bake in the toaster oven at 450°F (230°C, or gas mark 8) until the cheese is bubbly and starting to brown (about 5 minutes). Cut into wedges and devour, watching out for pizza burns!

If you don't have a toaster oven, you have a couple of options: You can make the pizza in a conventional oven, but it will take a while to get up to 450°F (230°C, gas mark 8). You can cook it in a dry skillet, like an open-faced quesadilla—but you won't flip it, of course! This will melt the cheese, especially if you cover the pan with a tilted lid, but the cheese won't brown. If I were doing it this way, I'd cook it until the cheese was just melting and then put the whole skillet under the broiler for a minute to brown the cheese. (Make sure your skillet has an ovenproof handle, if you decide to do this.) Or you could just put the pizza sauce and cheese on half of the tortilla and fold it over like a quesadilla.

Yield: 1 serving, with 16 grams of carbohydrates and 9 grams of fiber, for a total of 7 grams of usable carbs (you can drop it a little lower by using really low-carb pizza sauce) and 18 grams of protein.

Note: Ragu makes a good pizza sauce with no added sugar that's widely available. However, they also make one with sugar (corn syrup, actually), so read the label!

⊕ Not-Just-for-Breakfast Burrito

I know most people won't do this much cooking when they're trying to get out of the house in the morning. However, this makes a killer lunch or supper or even a hefty snack—and if you do want a really solid, incredibly yummy breakfast, be aware that I had this not only made but eaten well inside the 15-minute mark!

> 1 low-carb tortilla
>
> 2 ounces (55 g) shredded Monterey Jack cheese
>
> 2 scallions
>
> 1/4 ripe avocado
>
> 2 eggs
>
> 2 tablespoons (33 g) salsa
>
> 1 tablespoon (15 g) sour cream
>
> 1 tablespoon (1 g) chopped cilantro (optional, but mighty tasty)

Place the tortilla on a plate and spread the cheese over it. Place the plate in your microwave. Don't nuke it yet, though.

Slice the scallions and peel and slice the avocado.

Spray a medium-size skillet with nonstick cooking spray and put it over medium-high heat. Now take a second to go set your microwave for 60 seconds at 50 percent power. Start the microwave, come back, beat the eggs, pour them into the skillet, and scramble them until they're set. Turn off the heat under the pan.

Pull the tortilla with its melted cheese out of the microwave. Arrange the scrambled eggs down the middle and then top with the scallions, avocado, salsa, sour cream, and cilantro if you have some in the house. Fold as best you can—the burrito will be full to bursting!—and eat with the help of several napkins. Unbelievable!

Yield: 1 serving, with 22 grams of carbohydrates and 13 grams of fiber, for a total of 9 grams of usable carbs and 33 grams of protein.

✻ This burrito also packs 680 milligrams of potassium and 582 milligrams of calcium!

chapter three

15~Minute Burgers

When we first discussed this project, my editor, Holly, and I discussed recipes that simply wouldn't work for the 15-minute framework. Holly brought up meat loaves. "Hah!" I said. "I'll just make them as burgers."

And that's what I've done. Here, for your quick-cooking, low-carbing pleasure, is an astonishing variety of interesting burger recipes, not a few of which originated as high-carb meat loaf recipes.

All of these recipes assume that you have an electric tabletop grill—you know, the George Foreman kind of thing. Since these grills cook from both sides, they cook very rapidly. If you don't have one, no worries—there's no reason you can't cook these burgers in a skillet or even broil them—it'll just take an extra 5 minutes or so, and you'll have to flip them.

By the way, you'll find a number of burger recipes here that use pork. If you don't eat pork, I don't see any reason why ground turkey wouldn't work in these recipes. It would taste different, but should still taste good. If you do this, chop all of your other ingredients in a food processor and then add the ground turkey and pulse just long enough to combine.

⊕ Beef, Sausage, and Spinach Burgers

These are superb, and of course they have enough vegetables in them that you don't really have to eat anything else with them if you don't want to take the trouble—but some bagged Italian salad mix with Italian or Creamy Garlic dressing would sure go well!

1 pound (455 g) ground beef

1/2 pound (225 g) Italian sausage, hot or mild

1 package (10 ounces, or 280 g) chopped frozen spinach, thawed

1 teaspoon minced garlic or 2 cloves garlic, crushed

2 teaspoons Italian seasoning

1/2 teaspoon red pepper flakes

2 tablespoons (12 g) oat bran

1 egg

3 tablespoons (15 g) grated Parmesan cheese

1/2 teaspoon salt

1/2 cup (123 g) no-sugar-added spaghetti sauce

2 tablespoons (18 g) sliced ripe olives

Extra Parmesan cheese for topping

Preheat your electric tabletop grill.

Dump the ground beef, sausage, spinach, garlic, seasoning, red pepper, oat bran, egg, cheese, and salt into a big bowl. (If your Italian sausage came in casings—mine did—slit them and squeeze out the meat, discarding the casings.) Using clean hands, smoosh everything together very well; you want the flavors of the two meats completely blended.

Form into 5 burgers, each about 1 inch (2.5 cm) thick. Slap 'em on the electric grill and set a timer for 6 minutes.

While the burgers are cooking, combine the spaghetti sauce and olives in a micro-waveable bowl and nuke for 1 minute at 70 percent power.

When the stove timer goes off, stick a burger with a fork. If the juices run clear, they're done. If they're pink, give the burgers another minute. When they're cooked through, transfer them to serving plates, top each with the spaghetti sauce and olives, plus more Parmesan if you like, and serve.

Yield: 5 servings, each with 9 grams of carbohydrates and 3 grams of fiber, for a total of 6 grams of usable carbs and 26 grams of protein, not counting any extra Parmesan you may put on top.

✻ This recipe's a good source of calcium and vitamin A, too!

☉ Apple Sausage Burgers

Feel free to make these with turkey sausage, if you prefer.

> 1/2 medium onion, peeled and cut in a few chunks
>
> 1/2 Granny Smith or other crisp, tart apple, cut into a few chunks (no need to peel it)
>
> 1 1/2 pounds (680 g) bulk pork sausage, hot or mild
>
> 1 teaspoon dried thyme
>
> 1 teaspoon dried sage
>
> 1 teaspoon pepper

Preheat your electric tabletop grill.

Put the onion and apple in a food processor with the S-blade in place and pulse until they're chopped to a medium consistency. Add the sausage, thyme, sage, and pepper and pulse until it's all well-blended.

Form into 4 burger and put them on the grill. Cook for 7 minutes or until the juices run clear.

Yield: 4 servings, each with 7 grams of carbohydrates and 1 gram of fiber, for a total of 6 grams of usable carbs and 20 grams of protein.

⊕ Apple Cheddar Pork Burgers

What can I say? I think apples and pork are a terrific combination.

  1/2 Granny Smith or other crisp, tart apple, cut into a few chunks
    (no need to peel it)
  1/4 medium onion, peeled and cut into a couple of chunks
  1 pound (455 g) boneless pork loin, cut into 1 1/2-inch (3.8 cm) cubes
  2 tablespoons (12 g) oat bran
  1 egg
  1/2 teaspoon salt or Vege-Sal
  2 teaspoons prepared horseradish
  2 ounces (55 g) cheddar cheese, shredded

Preheat your electric tabletop grill.

Put the apple, onion, pork, oat bran, egg, salt or Voge-Sal, and horseradish in a food processor and pulse until the meat is ground and everything is well-blended. Add the cheese and pulse just long enough to blend it in—we're trying to keep some actual shreds of cheese here.

Form into 4 burgers and slap 'em on the grill. Cook for 7 minutes or until the juices run clear.

Yield: 4 servings, each with 5 grams of carbohydrates and 1 gram of fiber, for a total of 4 grams of usable carbs and 25 grams of protein.

⊕ Cranberry Burgers

Someone anonymously posted a recipe for burgers with cranberry jelly in them to the Internet. It was clearly high-carb, but it looked so tasty that I had to figure out a way to adapt it. Here it is! Don't panic at this list of ingredients because this really is quite quick and easy—you just dump stuff in the food processor and run it.

5 slices bacon

1 small onion, peeled and cut into chunks

1/3 cup (34 g) whole cranberries

2 cloves fresh garlic or 1 teaspoon minced garlic

1/4 green pepper, core and seeds removed, cut into a couple of chunks

1 stalk celery, cut into a few chunks

1 pound (455 g) ground beef

2 tablespoons (12 g) oat bran

1 egg

1/4 cup (6 g) Splenda

1/2 teaspoon grated gingerroot

5 ounces (140 g) cheddar cheese, in slices

First, begin cooking the bacon in the microwave using either a microwave bacon rack or a glass pie plate. In my microwave, 5 minutes on High (1 minute per slice) is about right, but microwave power varies.

Preheat your electric tabletop grill.

Put the onion, cranberries, garlic, pepper, and celery in your food processor with the S-blade in place and pulse to chop everything to a medium consistency. Add the ground beef, oat bran, egg, Splenda, and gingerroot and pulse again to combine. Form the mixture—it will be pretty soft—into 5 burgers. Put them on the grill and set a timer for 6 minutes.

While the burgers are cooking, go check the bacon. If it's still a little flabby, give it another minute or so; it should be crisp. Drain the bacon if needed and break each strip into 2 or 3 pieces to fit on top of the burgers.

When the 6 minutes are up, open your grill but do not remove the burgers. Arrange the bacon on the burgers and top each burger with cheddar cheese. Now, using a coffee mug or any other random, heat resistant kitchen object that's handy, prop the lid of your grill up so that it's above the burgers and close to, but not touching, the cheese. Let the burgers cook for another minute or two to melt the cheese and then serve.

Yield: 5 servings, each with 8 grams of carbohydrates and 1 gram of fiber, for a total of 7 grams of usable carbs and 42 grams of protein.

Note: Cranberries are one of the very few foods that are still strictly seasonal— they're only available in the fall. However, they freeze brilliantly; just toss a plastic bag of them in the deep freeze, and it will live there happily for months. So pick up a few extra bags during the Thanksgiving shopping season and enjoy these burgers all year long.

⊕ Ham and Pork Burgers

These are sort of plain and simple, but my husband loves them. This is a good recipe to help you use up leftover ham, should you have any on hand—but of course, you can also buy a chunk of precooked ham at the grocery store.

> 1/2 pound (225 g) cooked ham, cut into chunks
> 3/4 pound (340 g) boneless pork loin, cut into chunks
> 2 tablespoons (12 g) oat bran
> 2 tablespoons (28 ml) heavy cream
> 1 egg
> 1/2 teaspoon pepper

Preheat your electric tabletop grill.

Plunk the ham, pork loin, oat bran, cream, egg, and pepper in a food processor with the S-blade in place and pulse until the meat is finely ground. Form into 4 burgers and put them in the grill. Cook for 6 to 7 minutes and serve.

Yield: 4 servings, each with no more than 5 grams of carbohydrates (less, if you use really low-carb ham) and 1 gram of fiber, for a total of no more than 4 grams of usable carbs and 28 grams of protein.

☉ Orange Lamb Burgers

Don't bother grinding your own lamb in your food processor; I tried this, and it came out a bit gristly. Buy ground lamb, instead. If you can't find ground lamb at your grocery store, ask the nice meat guy.

1/4 large sweet red onion

2 cloves garlic or 1 teaspoon minced garlic

1 pound (455 g) ground lamb

1 teaspoon ground cumin

1 1/2 tablespoons (23 ml) soy sauce

2 teaspoons grated orange zest

2 tablespoons (28 ml) orange juice

2 tablespoons (2 g) chopped cilantro

1/4 teaspoon salt

1/2 teaspoon pepper

Preheat your electric tabletop grill.

Either chop the red onion and the garlic to a medium-fine consistency in your food processor using the S-blade or cut 'em up with a knife. Then put them and the lamb, cumin, soy sauce, orange zest, orange juice, cilantro, salt, and pepper in a big bowl. Using clean hands, smoosh everything together until it's all very well blended. Form the mixture into 4 burgers and put them on the grill. Cook for 7 minutes and serve.

Yield: 4 servings, each with 3 grams of carbohydrates, a trace of fiber, and 20 grams of protein.

⊕ Mediterranean Lamb Burgers

This is about as upscale as a cheeseburger can get. My husband, who generally prefers beef to lamb, thought these were great.

> 1/4 medium onion
>
> 2 tablespoons (7 g) sun-dried tomatoes
>
> 1 pound (455 g) ground lamb
>
> 1 tablespoon (15 g) jarred pesto sauce
>
> 1 tablespoon (10 g) chopped garlic
>
> 1/4 teaspoon pepper
>
> 1/2 teaspoon salt or Vege-Sal
>
> 2 tablespoons (18 g) pine nuts
>
> 3 ounces (85 g) chèvre (goat) cheese

Preheat your electric tabletop grill; I set mine to 350°F (180°C).

Chop your onion and if your sun-dried tomatoes are in halves rather than pre-chopped, chop them up, too. Heck, even if they're prechopped, chop them a little more. Throw these things in a mixing bowl.

Add the ground lamb, pesto, garlic, pepper, and salt. Use clean hands to squish it all together until it's well-mixed. Form into three patties and throw them in the grill. Set a timer for 5 minutes.

While the burgers are cooking, toast your pine nuts until they're touched with gold.

When your burgers are done, plate them, crumble an ounce (28 g) of chèvre over each one, sprinkle with pine nuts, and then serve.

Yield: 3 servings, each with 578 calories, 47 grams fat, 33 grams protein, 4 grams carbohydrate, 1 gram dietary fiber, and 3 grams usable carb.

⊕Thai Burgers

Boy are these good! If you can't find fish sauce, you can substitute soy sauce and this will still taste fine.

1 1/2 pounds (680 g) boneless pork loin, cut into chunks

1 1/2 teaspoons lemon juice

1 tablespoon (16 g) chili garlic paste

1 clove garlic or 1/2 teaspoon minced garlic

4 scallions, with the roots and the tops cut off
(leave the crisp part of the green!)

1 can 4 ounces, or (15 g) mushrooms, drained

1 tablespoon (15 ml) fish sauce

2 tablespoons (2 g) fresh cilantro

3 tablespoons (45 ml) lime juice

1/2 cup (115 g) mayonnaise (100 ml)

Preheat your electric tabletop grill.

Put the pork loin, lemon juice, garlic paste, garlic, scallions, mushrooms, fish sauce, and cilantro in a food processor with the S-blade in place. Pulse until the meat is finely ground and everything is well-combined. Form the mixture into 6 burgers and put them on the grill. Cook for 6 to 7 minutes.

While the burgers are cooking, stir the lime juice (bottled works fine) into the mayonnaise. When the burgers are done, top each one with a dollop of the lime mayonnaise and serve.

Yield: 6 servings, each with 4 grams of carbohydrates and 1 gram of fiber, for a total of 3 grams of usable carbs and 24 grams of protein.

⊕ Banh Mi Burgers

I saw a recipe for a Vietnamese meatball sandwich and thought, "I could make that into burgers." So I did. For a full meal, make the *Hot and Sweet Mostly Asian Slaw* on page 254 and serve the burgers and sauce on top of the slaw. But these are tasty even without the slaw!

5 scallions, divided

1/4 (15 g) cup fresh basil leaves

1 pound (455 g) ground pork

2 teaspoons chopped garlic

1 tablespoon (20 g) fish sauce

1 tablespoon (20 g) Sriracha chili sauce

1 tablespoon (1.5 g) Splenda, or its equivalent in sweetness

1 teaspoon salt

1 teaspoon pepper

1/3 cup (75 g) mayonnaise

1 tablespoon (20 g) Sriracha chili sauce

Preheat electric tabletop grill. If you can choose temperature settings on yours, use 350°F (180°C).

Cut the root and any limp greens off the scallions, whack them into a few pieces, and throw three of them into your food processor with the S-blade in place. (Reserve the other two.) Throw in the basil, too. Pulse until they're finely chopped together.

Now add ingredients from the pork through the pepper and run the processor until it's all well-blended.

Make the pork mixture into three patties and put them in the grill. Set a timer for 6 to 8 minutes.

Quickly wash out your food processor and reassemble with the S-blade in place. Put the remaining scallions in there and pulse to chop. Now add the mayo and chili sauce and run to blend.

When the burgers are done, serve with the sauce.

Yield: 3 servings, each with 597 calories, 53 grams fat, 27 grams protein, 5 grams carbohydrate, 1 gram dietary fiber, and 4 grams usable carb.

⏱ Luau Burgers

Again, all those ingredients make this look intimidating, but it's really just a matter of assembling everything in the food processor and chopping it together.

  1 pound (455 g) boneless pork loin

  1/4 medium onion, cut into chunks

  1/2 green pepper, cut into chunks

  1 1/2 teaspoons grated gingerroot

  1/2 teaspoon minced garlic or 1 clove garlic, crushed

  1 tablespoon (15 ml) soy sauce

  1 egg

  1/4 cup (60 g) crushed pork rinds, plain or barbeque flavor

  1/2 teaspoon pepper

  1/2 teaspoon salt

  1/4 cup (60 g) canned crushed pineapple in unsweetened juice

  1 tablespoon (15 g) tomato sauce

  1/2 teaspoon blackstrap molasses

  1/2 teaspoon Splenda

  1/2 teaspoon spicy brown mustard

Preheat your electric tabletop grill.

Place the pork, onion, pepper, gingerroot, garlic, soy sauce, egg, pork rinds, pepper, and salt in a food processor with the S-blade in place. (You'll need a full-size food processor; this overwhelmed my little one!) Pulse until the meat is finely ground. Add the pineapple and pulse to mix.

Form into 5 burgers—the mixture will be quite soft—and slap them on the grill. Set a timer for 6 minutes.

While the burgers are cooking, mix together the tomato sauce, molasses, Splenda, and mustard. When the 6 minutes are up, open the grill, spread the tomato sauce mixture evenly over the burgers, and then close the grill and cook for 1 more minute. Serve.

Yield: 5 servings, each with 5 grams of carbohydrates and 1 gram of fiber, for a total of 4 grams of usable carbs and 22 grams of protein.

✴ These are low calorie, too! Just 178 calories per serving.

☉ Chili Burgers

Here's all the long-simmered flavor of chili in a fast-and-easy burger.

> 1 pound (455 g) ground beef
>
> 1 cup (241 g) canned tomatoes with green chilies
>
> 1/2 medium onion, finely minced
>
> 2 cloves garlic, crushed
>
> 1 tablespoon (8 g) chili powder
>
> 2 tablespoons (30 g) crushed barbecue-flavor pork rinds
>
> 1 tablespoon (16 g) tomato paste
>
> 1 tablespoon (18 g) salt or Vege-Sal
>
> 4 ounces (115 g) cheddar cheese, sliced
>
> Sour cream (optional)

Preheat your electric tabletop grill.

Plunk the beef, tomatoes, onion, garlic, chili powder, pork rinds, tomato paste, and salt into a bowl and using clean hands, smoosh it all together until everything is thoroughly combined. Form this mixture into 4 patties, put them on the grill, and cook for 5 minutes.

When the 5 minutes are up, open your grill but do not remove the burgers. Top each with a slice of cheddar cheese and use whatever heatproof kitchen object you have on hand to prop the lid of the grill open slightly for a minute or so. Let the cheese melt and serve with a dollop of sour cream, if you like.

Yield: 4 servings, each with 6 grams of carbohydrates and 1 gram of fiber, for a total of 5 grams of usable carbs and 28 grams of protein. Add 1 gram of carbs and 1 gram of protein if you use the sour cream.

Variation: These would be great with a big, simple green salad with cucumbers, green peppers, and a few tomato slices, tossed with ranch dressing.

⊕Crunchy Peking Burgers

½ cup (62 g) canned water chestnuts, drained

2 scallions

1 pound (455 g) ground beef

¼ cup (60 ml) soy sauce

2 tablespoons (28 ml) dry sherry

1 teaspoon Splenda

1 teaspoon minced garlic or 2 cloves garlic, crushed

½ teaspoon grated gingerroot

Sauce

1 ½ tablespoons (30 g) low-sugar apricot preserves

1 teaspoon soy sauce

¼ teaspoon grated gingerroot

Preheat your electric tabletop grill.

Chop the water chestnuts a bit and slice the scallions. Put them in a mixing bowl with all the other burger ingredients and using clean hands, mix them well. Form into 4 burgers and put them on the grill. Cook for 5 minutes.

While the burgers are cooking, mix together the preserves, soy sauce, and gingerroot in a small dish. When the burgers are done, top each with a teaspoon of sauce and serve.

Yield: 4 servings, each with 7 grams of carbohydrates and 1 gram of fiber, for a total of 6 grams of usable carbs and 20 grams of protein.

⊕ Many-Pepper Burgers

Burger recipes don't get much simpler than this one!

> 1 pound (455 g) ground beef
>
> 2 1/2 tablespoons (18 g) *Many-Pepper Steak Seasoning* (see page 302)

Preheat your electric tabletop grill.

In a mixing bowl, use clean hands to mix the ground beef and seasoning together. Form into 3 or 4 burgers and cook them on the grill for 5 to 6 minutes.

Yield: 3 or 4 servings. Assuming 3 servings, each will have 1 gram of carbohydrates, a trace of fiber, and 25 grams of protein.

⊕ All-American Turkey Burgers

How spicy these are will depend on what sort of hot sauce you use. They're really good with coleslaw. (See the recipe for *Coleslaw Dressing* on page 299).

> 1 pound (455 g) ground turkey
>
> 1/2 medium onion, finely chopped
>
> 1 stalk celery, finely chopped
>
> 1 teaspoon dried thyme
>
> 1 tablespoon (16 g) low-carbohydrate barbecue sauce, homemade
>   or purchased
>
> 1 teaspoon hot sauce
>
> 2 teaspoons Worcestershire sauce

Preheat your electric tabletop grill.

Simply combine everything and form the mixture into 3 burgers. Throw them on the grill, cook for 5 minutes, and serve.

Yield: 3 servings. The carb count will vary a bit depending on what barbecue sauce you use, but it should be in the neighborhood of 4 grams of carbohydrates and 1 gram of fiber, for a total of 3 grams of usable carbs and 27 grams of protein.

☉ Wing Burgers

Why are these *Wing Burgers*? Because this combination of seasonings was inspired by the coating of *Heroin Wings*, the very first recipe in my first cookbook, *500 Low-Carb Recipes*, and a perennial favorite. It's no big surprise that the flavors are great in burgers, too.

> 1 pound (455 g) ground chuck
>
> 1/2 cup (50 g) grated Parmesan cheese
>
> 1 tablespoon (1 g) dried parsley
>
> 1/2 tablespoon Italian seasoning
>
> 1 teaspoon paprika
>
> 1/4 teaspoon salt or Vege-Sal
>
> 1/4 teaspoon pepper
>
> 1 egg

This is so simple! Start your electric table-top grill preheating to 350°F (180°C). Plunk all the ingredients into a big mixing bowl and use clean hands to squish them up until it's all well-blended. Make three patties and throw them on the grill for five minutes. If you want to top them with something—though they're good as-is—skip the ketchup and use a little no-sugar-added pizza sauce.

Yield: 3 servings, each with 488 calories, 37 grams fat, 34 grams protein, 2 grams carbohydrate, trace dietary fiber, and 2 grams usable carb.

☺ Salmon Patties

That Nice Boy I Married said these were the best salmon patties he'd ever had. And this recipe calls for stuff that keeps and so is likely to be hanging around the house, making it extra convenient.

> 2 ounces (55 g) pork rinds
>
> 1/2 medium onion
>
> 1/4 cup (15 g) parsley
>
> 1 can (14 ounces, or 390 g) salmon
>
> 2 eggs
>
> 1 1/2 teaspoons brown mustard
>
> 1 teaspoon chopped garlic
>
> 2 tablespoons (16 g) coconut flour
>
> 4 tablespoons (55 g) butter

Put your big, heavy skillet over medium-low heat and get it warming.

Throw the pork rinds in your food processor and pulse until they're reduced to crumbs. Dump them half of them in a mixing bowl and half on a plate.

Now throw the onion and parsley in the food processor and chop those together, too. Add them to the mixing bowl.

Add the canned salmon to the bowl and break it up, picking out any bones. Add the eggs, mustard, garlic, and coconut flour and work everything together well.

Throw half the butter in the skillet and slosh it around as it melts. Now make the salmon mixture into four patties and coat them on both sides with the reserved pork rind crumbs. Fry in the butter until they're well-browned on the bottom. Add the rest of the butter to the skillet as you flip them and brown the other side. Serve!

Yield: 4 servings, each with 391 calories, 25 grams fat, 33 grams protein, 7 grams carbohydrate, 4 grams dietary fiber, and 3 grams usable carb.

15~Minute Poultry

You'll find that most of these recipes depend upon the ubiquitous boneless, skinless chicken breast. There's a reason for this: It's nearly impossible to cook chicken on the bone in 15 minutes or less! And even with boneless, skinless chicken breasts, it's helpful, in a fair number of recipes, to pound them a little to make them thinner and an even thickness all over. This is very easy to do and takes no more than 15 to 30 seconds per breast—time well spent if it cuts 5 minutes off the cooking time. Once you've beaten a chicken breast flat a few times, you'll wonder why you've never done it before.

⊕ Lemon Chicken

This Vietnamese-influenced dish has a subtle lemon-garlic flavor that combines beautifully with the spicy tart-sweet dipping sauce. And even including making the dipping sauce, this is done within our 15-minute time limit!

> 1 1/2 pounds (680 g) boneless, skinless chicken breast
>
> 1 tablespoon (15 ml) plus 1 teaspoon (5 ml) lemon juice
>
> 2 teaspoons garlic
>
> 1 tablespoon (1.5 g) plus 1 teaspoon (0.5 g) Splenda
>
> 2 teaspoons fish sauce (nuoc mam)
>
> 1/2 teaspoon pepper
>
> Oil
>
> *Nuoc Cham* dipping sauce (see page 292)

First, put the chicken breasts, one at a time, in a heavy zipper-lock bag and use any blunt object available to beat them until they're 1/2 inch (1.3 cm) thick all over. Put them on a plate after they're beaten into submission.

Mix together the lemon juice, garlic, Splenda, fish sauce, and pepper and pour the mixture evenly over the chicken breasts, turning them to make sure all sides get coated. Heat a tablespoon or two (15 to 28 ml) of oil in a heavy skillet over medium-high heat and add the chicken breasts. Sauté for 4 to 5 minutes per side or until cooked through.

While the chicken is sautéing, throw together the *Nuoc Cham*—this takes maybe two minutes!

In the last minute or so, pour the lemon juice mixture remaining on the plate into the skillet, turning the breasts to once again make sure both sides are coated. Heat for 1 minute and remove to serving plates. Serve with a little pool or dish of *Nuoc Cham* to dip bites of chicken in.

Yield: 4 servings, each with 6 grams of carbohydrate, a trace of fiber, and 38 grams of protein.

⊕ Singing Chicken

This is another Vietnamese dish, and it is definitely for those who enjoy breathing fire. I'm a big fan of hot food, and this dish had me sweating by halfway through the meal. Delicious! It's droccoli goes nicely with this.

2 to 3 tablespoons (28 to 45 ml) vegetable oil, preferably peanut

1 tablespoon (8 g) grated gingerroot

1 teaspoon minced garlic or 2 cloves garlic, crushed

1 1/2 pounds (680 g) boneless, skinless chicken breast,
   cut crosswise into thin slices*

2 tablespoons (3 g) Splenda

1/4 cup (60 ml) soy sauce

1 teaspoon fish sauce (nuoc mam)

3/4 cup (175 ml) dry white wine

1 fresh jalapeño, or 2 or 3 little red chilies, finely minced

1 teaspoon pepper

Guar or xanthan

* This is easiest if the meat is half-frozen.

Have the chicken sliced, the ingredients measured, the pepper minced, and everything standing by and ready to go before starting to cook—once you start stir-frying, this goes very quickly.

Put a wok or heavy skillet over high heat. Add the oil, let it heat for a minute or so, and then add the ginger and garlic. Stir for 1 minute to flavor the oil. Add the chicken, and stir-fry for 1 to 2 minutes. Add the Splenda, soy sauce, fish sauce, white wine, jalapeño, and pepper, stirring often, for 7 to 8 minutes or until the chicken is cooked through. Thicken pan juices very slightly with guar or xanthan and serve.

Yield: 3 or 4 servings. Assuming 4 servings, each will have 4 grams of carbohydrates, a trace of fiber, and 39 grams of protein.

☉ Crispy Skillet BBQ Chicken

Add some slaw made from bagged coleslaw mix, and supper is served.

> 1 1/2 pounds (680 g) boneless, skinless chicken breast
>
> Sprinkle-on barbecue dry rub or "soul" seasoning
>
> 1/2 cup (120 g) crushed barbecue-flavor pork rinds
>
> 2 tablespoons (28 ml) oil

One at a time, pound the chicken breasts until they're about 1/2 inch (1.3 cm) thick all over. If necessary, cut the breasts into 4 servings. Sprinkle both sides of each piece liberally with the seasoning. Then sprinkle each side of each serving with 1 tablespoon (15 g) of the pork rind crumbs and press them onto the surface with a clean palm.

Heat the oil in a large, heavy-bottomed skillet over medium-high heat. Add the chicken breasts and sauté for 5 to 6 minutes per side or until crispy and cooked through. Serve. This is great with any sort of salad or coleslaw as a side.

Yield: 4 servings. This has no carbs to speak of (maybe a tiny trace from the seasoning), no fiber, and 44 grams of protein per serving.

☉ Aegean Chicken

The minute I told my sister about this, she started hounding me for the recipe.

> 1 1/2 pounds (680 g) boneless, skinless chicken breast
>
> 1/4 cup (60 ml) olive oil
>
> 4 ounces (115 g) kasseri cheese, sliced
>
> 8 tablespoons (64 g) tapenade
>
> 1/4 cup (60 ml) dry white wine
>
> 2 cloves garlic

One at a time, pound the chicken breasts till they're 1/4 inch (6 mm) thick all over. Cut the breasts into 6 servings, if necessary. Sauté them in the olive oil over medium-high heat. When they're turning golden on the bottom, turn them and lay the slices of kasseri over them. Let them cook another 2 to 3 minutes or until the cheese is starting to melt. Spread the tapenade over the breasts and add the wine to the skillet. Let the whole thing cook for another minute or two, just to warm the tapenade and make sure the chicken is cooked through. Remove the chicken to serving plates, add the garlic to the wine left in the skillet, stir the whole thing and let it boil for a minute or so, and pour it over the chicken before serving.

Yield: 6 servings, each with just 2 grams of carbohydrates, a trace of fiber, and 40 grams of protein.

⊕ Cashew Crusted Chicken

Since cashews are a relatively high-carb nut, this is just a light coating—but very flavorful. You can find raw cashews at most health food stores.

> 2/3 cup (93 g) raw cashew pieces
>
> 1/4 teaspoon salt
>
> 1/2 teaspoon pepper
>
> 1/4 teaspoon paprika
>
> 1 1/2 pounds (680 g) boneless, skinless chicken breast
>
> 1 egg
>
> 2 to 3 tablespoons (28 to 42 g) butter

First, put the cashew pieces in a food processor with the S-blade in place and grind them to a fine texture. Dump them out onto a plate and add the salt, pepper, and paprika, mixing the whole thing well. Set aside.

Pound the chicken breasts until they're 1/2 inch (1.3 cm) thick all over. Cut into 4 servings if necessary.

Break the egg into another plate with a rim around it. (A pie plate would work well.) Now, dip each chicken breast piece into the egg, then into the cashew mixture, coating both sides.

Melt the butter in a heavy skillet over medium to medium-high heat and add the chicken. Sauté until it's golden on both sides and cooked through, about 5 minutes per side.

Yield: 4 servings, each with 6 grams of carbohydrates and 1 gram of fiber, for a total of 5 grams of usable carbs and 33 grams of protein.

☉ Almond Chicken with Gorgonzola Cream Sauce

This dish is simply fantastic—lush and creamy and decadent. It's just fantastic. Do pound the chicken out thin enough, though, or it'll take an extra few minutes.

1 pound (455 g) boneless, skinless chicken breast

1 tablespoon (14 g) butter

1 tablespoon (15 ml) olive oil

1 cup (112 g) almond meal

2 tablespoons (16 g) coconut flour

1/2 teaspoon salt or Vege-Sal

1/4 teaspoon pepper

1 teaspoon ground sage

1 egg

1 tablespoon (15 ml) water

1/4 cup (60 ml) dry white wine

1 cup (235 ml) heavy cream

1/2 cup (60 g) crumbled gorgonzola cheese

salt and pepper

2 tablespoons (3 g) minced parsley

Set your big, heavy skillet over medium heat.

Using a blunt, heavy object, beat your chicken breast out to 1/4 to 1/3 inch (6 mm to 8 mm) thick. Cut into four portions.

On a plate with a rim, combine the almond meal, coconut flour, salt, pepper, and sage. On another plate, beat up the egg with the water.

Add the butter and olive oil to the skillet and slosh them around.

Dip each piece of chicken in the egg on both sides, then the almond meal mixture. Lay them in the skillet and cover with a tilted lid.

While the chicken is cooking, measure out the wine, cream, and gorgonzola.

Okay, chicken's golden on one side. Flip it and cook the other, again, with the tilted lid over it.

When the chicken's done, plate it and keep it warm.

Add the wine to the skillet and crank the heat up to high. Boil it down for a minute and then add the cream and the gorgonzola. Let the sauce boil hard, stirring constantly until it's reduced and thickened a bit. You can add a little guar, xanthan, or glucomannan if you like. Salt and pepper the sauce, spoon it over the chicken, top with parsley, and serve.

Yield: 4 servings, each with 645 calories, 43 grams fat, 46 grams protein, 18 grams carbohydrate, 4 grams dietary fiber, and 14 grams usable carb.

⊕ Chicken Breast Italiano

This dish is ridiculously easy, especially considering how good it tastes! It's great with one of the cauliflower "risottos" as a side dish (see page 234 and 235).

> 1 1/2 pounds (680 g) boneless, skinless chicken breast
>
> 2 tablespoons (28 ml) olive oil
>
> 1/3 cup (80 ml) bottled Italian salad dressing

In a heavy-bottomed skillet, sauté the chicken breasts in the olive oil over medium heat. Cover them while they're cooking and turn them after 6 to 7 minutes. When both sides are golden and the chicken is cooked most of the way through, add the Italian dressing, turn the breasts to coat both sides, and let the whole thing cook for another 2 to 3 minutes before serving.

Yield: 4 servings, each with 2 grams of carbohydrates, no fiber, and 38 grams of protein.

⊕ Chicken Tenders

This is good for when you're having fast-food cravings or the kids are nagging for "normal" food. You really can make these in 15 minutes—because the pieces are small, they cook very quickly.

> 1 pound (455 g) boneless, skinless chicken breast
>
> 1 egg
>
> 1 tablespoon (15 ml) water
>
> 3/4 cup (94 g) low-carb bake mix
>
> 1/2 teaspoon salt
>
> 1/4 teaspoon pepper
>
> 1/3 cup (80 ml) oil

Cut the chicken breasts into pieces about 1 inch (2.5 cm) wide and 2 inches (5 cm) long. Beat the egg with the water in a bowl. On a plate, combine the bake mix with the salt and pepper. Heat the oil in a heavy skillet over medium-high heat.

Dip each chicken piece in the egg wash, then roll it in the seasoned bake mix, and drop it in the hot oil. Fry these until golden all over and serve with one of the dipping sauces in the *Condiments, Sauces, Dressings, and Seasonings* chapter (see page 289).

Yield: 4 servings, each with 5 grams of carbohydrates and 2 grams of fiber, for a total of 3 grams of usable carbs (exclusive of the dipping sauces) and 40 grams of protein.

☉ Seriously Spicy Citrus Chicken

You could cut back on the red pepper flakes if you'd like to make Moderately Spicy Citrus Chicken.

1 1/2 pounds (680 g) boneless, skinless chicken breast

1/4 cup (60 ml) olive oil

1/2 cup (120 ml) lime juice

1/4 cup (60 ml) lemon juice

1 tablespoon (4 g) plus 1 teaspoon (1 g) red pepper flakes

1 tablespoon (6 g) plus 1 teaspoon (2 g) minced garlic

1 tablespoon (8 g) plus 1 teaspoon (3 g) grated gingerroot

1/4 cup (6 g) Splenda

4 scallions, finely sliced

2 tablespoons (2 g) chopped cilantro

Cut the chicken into 4 servings, if necessary. Sauté the chicken in the olive oil over medium-high heat, with a tilted lid. While it's sautéing, mix together the lime juice, lemon juice, red pepper flakes, garlic, gingerroot, and Splenda. After the chicken has turned golden on both sides (about 4 to 5 minutes per side), pour the lime juice mixture into the skillet and turn the breasts over to coat both sides. Sauté for another 2 to 3 minutes on each side and then move the chicken to serving plates, scraping the liquid from the pan over the chicken. Scatter sliced scallions and chopped cilantro over each portion and serve.

Yield: 4 servings, each with 8 grams of carbohydrates and 1 gram of fiber, for a total of 7 grams of usable carbs and 32 grams of protein.

⊕ Lemon-Herb Chicken Breast

This dish is simple and classic and summery.

> 1 teaspoon chopped garlic
>
> 1/2 cup (120 ml) olive oil
>
> 1 pound (455 g) boneless, skinless chicken breast
>
> salt and pepper
>
> 1/4 cup (10 g) minced fresh basil
>
> 2 tablespoons (5 g) minced fresh parsley
>
> 2 lemons
>
> 2 tablespoons (28 ml) water

Put the garlic in a measuring cup and pour the olive oil over it. Let it sit.

Give a skillet a squirt of nonstick cooking spray and put it over a high burner.

Now grab your chicken and a blunt, heavy object and pound your breast out to an even 1/2 inch (1.3 cm) thickness. Cut into three portions and salt and pepper it on both sides.

Pour half or so of the garlicky olive oil into your now-hot skillet, slosh it around, and throw in your chicken. Cover it with a tilted lid and let it cook for 3 to 4 minutes.

Mince your basil and parsley. Also roll your lemon under your palm, pressing down firmly. This will help it render more juice.

Your chicken should be golden on the bottom now; flip it! Re-cover with the tilted lid and give it another 3 to 4 minutes. In the meantime, slice your lemon in half and flick out the seeds with the tip of a knife.

When your chicken is golden on both sides, squeeze one of the lemons over it. Flip it to coat both sides, turn the burner down to medium low, and re-cover with that tilted lid. Let it cook until it's done through.

Plate your chicken and then add the water and the juice of the other lemon to the skillet. Stir it all around with a fork, scraping up the tasty brown bits, and then pour this over the chicken. Top with the herbs and a last drizzle of garlic olive oil and then serve.

Yield: 3 servings, each with 508 calories, 40 grams fat, 34 grams protein, 5 grams carbohydrate, 1 gram dietary fiber, and 4 grams usable carb.

◌ Apricot-Bourbon Chicken

This is amazing—as good as anything I've ever had in a fancy restaurant—yet it's fast enough to make on a weeknight after work! I like the *Saffron "Rice"* (see page 237) as a side with this.

> 2 pounds (900 g) boneless, skinless chicken breasts
>
> 3 tablespoons (42 g) butter
>
> 1/2 cup (55 g) chopped pecans
>
> 1/4 cup (80 g) low-sugar apricot preserves
>
> 1/4 cup (60 ml) bourbon
>
> 2 tablespoons (31 g) plain tomato sauce
>
> 2 teaspoons spicy brown or Dijon mustard
>
> 1/2 teaspoon minced garlic or 1 clove garlic, crushed
>
> 1/4 cup (40 g) minced onion
>
> 3 scallions, thinly sliced

First, pound the chicken breasts until they're 1/2 inch (1.3 cm) thick all over and cut into 6 portions. Brown them in 2 tablespoons (28 g) of butter in a large, heavy skillet over high heat.

While the breasts are browning, melt the last tablespoon (14 g) of butter in a small, heavy skillet and stir in the pecans. Stir them over medium-high heat for a few minutes until they begin to turn golden. Turn off the heat (and if yours is an electric stove, remove from the burner to prevent scorching) and reserve.

Stir together the preserves, bourbon, tomato sauce, mustard, garlic, and onion. When the chicken is light golden on both sides, pour this mixture into the skillet. Turn the chicken over once or twice to coat both sides with the sauce. Cover with a tilted lid and let it simmer for about 5 minutes or until cooked through.

Serve with the sauce spooned over each portion and top each with the toasted pecans and sliced scallions.

Yield: 6 servings, each with 7 grams of carbohydrates and 1 gram of fiber, for a total of 6 grams of usable carbs and 35 grams of protein.

☉ Chicken Breasts L'Orange

Chicken combines so well with all sorts of fruit flavors, and this dish is sure to be a hit with the whole family.

1 1/2 pounds (680 g) boneless, skinless chicken breast

1/4 cup (60 ml) oil

1/3 cup (80 ml) orange juice

2 tablespoons (3 g) Splenda

2 teaspoons cider vinegar

1/4 teaspoon blackstrap molasses

1 teaspoon spicy brown or Dijon mustard

1 teaspoon minced garlic or 2 cloves garlic, crushed

Salt and pepper

Cut the chicken breasts into 4 portions and brown them in the oil in a large, heavy skillet over high heat. While that's happening, mix together the orange juice, Splenda, vinegar, molasses, mustard, and garlic.

When the chicken is light golden on both sides, add the orange juice mixture to the skillet. Simmer the chicken for another 7 to 8 minutes, turning once. Salt and pepper to taste and serve.

Yield: 4 servings, each with 4 grams of carbohydrates, a trace of fiber, and 38 grams of protein.

☉ Chicken with Asparagus and Gruyère

1 1/2 pounds (680 g) boneless, skinless chicken breast

1 tablespoon (14 g) butter

1 pound (455 g) asparagus

1 tablespoon (15 ml) dry white wine

1 tablespoon (15 ml) lemon juice

Salt and pepper

4 ounces (115 g) gruyère cheese, thinly sliced

First, pound the chicken breasts until they're 1/4 inch (6 mm) thick all over. Cut into 4 portions.

Melt the butter in a large, heavy skillet over medium-high heat and start browning the chicken.

While that's happening, snap the ends off the asparagus where they break naturally. Put the asparagus in a microwaveable casserole or lay it in a glass pie plate. Add a couple of tablespoons (28 ml) of water and cover. (Use plastic wrap or a plate to cover if you're using a pie plate.) Microwave on High for 3 to 4 minutes.

When the chicken is golden on both sides, add the wine and the lemon juice to the skillet and turn the chicken breasts to coat both sides. Salt and pepper lightly. Turn the burner to medium-low heat and let the chicken continue to cook until the asparagus is done microwaving.

Remove the asparagus from the microwave and drain. Lay the asparagus spears over the chicken, dividing equally between the portions. Cover each with gruyère and cover the skillet with a tilted lid. Continue cooking a few minutes, just until the cheese is melted. Serve.

Yield: 4 servings, each with 3 grams of carbohydrates and 1 gram of fiber, for a total of 2 grams of usable carbs and 38 grams of protein.

⊕ Creamy Chicken and Noodles in a Bowl

This is as good a make-it-in-the-bowl recipe as I've ever come up with, and it's quite filling. I had this cooked and eaten before the timer beeped for 15 minutes.

> 1 package tofu shirataki, fettuccini width
>
> 1/4 cup (45 g) jarred roasted red peppers, drained and diced
>
> 5 kalamata olives, pitted and chopped
>
> 1 scallion, sliced, including the crisp part of the green shoot
>
> 1 tablespoon (4 g) minced fresh parsley
>
> 3 tablespoons (38 g) whipped cream cheese with chives and onions
>
> 3 ounces (85 g) precooked chicken breast strips—Mine had Southwestern seasoning.
>
> salt and pepper to taste

Snip open the packet of shirataki, drain and rinse them, and throw them in a microwaveable bowl. Nuke them on high for 90 seconds.

While that's happening, drain and dice your roasted red peppers.

When the microwave beeps, drain the shirataki again. Put it back in for another 90 seconds.

Pit your kalamatas—just squish them with your thumb and pick the pits out—then chop them up. Slice your scallion and chop your parsely, too.

Drain your noodles one last time. Now add the cream cheese and chicken breast strips and nuke it for just 30 more seconds.

When it comes out, throw in the peppers, olives, scallions, and parsley. Stir it up until the cheese melts, salt and pepper to taste, and devour!

Yield: 1 serving with 285 calories, 22 grams fat, 16 grams protein, 5 grams carbohydrate, 1 gram dietary fiber, and 4 grams usable carb.

⊕ Parmesan Chicken Breasts

Those of you who bought my first cookbook, *500 Low-Carb Recipes*, will recognize this recipe as being quite similar to *Heroin Wings*. However, *Heroin Wings* take well over an hour, and this is quite quick.

  1 ½ pounds (680 g) boneless, skinless chicken breast

  1 cup (100 g) grated Parmesan cheese*

  4 teaspoons (8 g) dried oregano

  1 teaspoon garlic powder

  1 teaspoon paprika

  1 teaspoon pepper

  2 eggs

  4 tablespoons (55 g) butter

* Use the cheap stuff in the round, green shaker for this.

Pound the chicken breasts till they're ¼ inch (6 mm) thick and cut into 6 portions. Set aside.

Combine the cheese with the oregano, garlic, paprika, and pepper on a plate. On another plate or in a shallow bowl, beat the eggs. Dip the chicken in the egg and then the cheese mixture, coating both sides well.

Melt the butter in a heavy skillet over medium-low heat (higher heat will scorch the cheese) and sauté for 4 to 5 minutes per side or until cooked through.

Yield: 6 servings, each with 2 grams of carbohydrates and 1 gram of fiber, for a total of 1 gram of usable carbs and 33 grams of protein.

⏱ Buffalo Chicken Breast

Wow! Pecan crusted chicken is cooked in butter, topped with Buffalo sauce, and served with the traditional blue cheese dressing. How could you not love it? You could throw in some celery sticks if you wanted to be really classical about it. You could also simplify by using bottled Buffalo sauce, but making it is a snap.

1 1/2 pounds (680 g) boneless, skinless chicken breast

1 cup (110 g) ground pecans

2 tablespoons (16 g) coconut flour

1 teaspoon salt

1/2 teaspoon pepper

1 egg

1 tablespoon (15 ml) water

1 stick butter, divided

1/4 cup (60 ml) Louisiana-style hot sauce—Frank's Red Hot is the canonical
   sauce for this, but Tabasco or any other Louisiana-style sauce will do.

8 tablespoons (120 g) blue cheese salad dressing—to serve

Pound the chicken out 1/4 inch (6 mm) thick and cut into 4 servings.

Put your big, heavy skillet over medium heat.

I started with purchased pecan meal, but if you don't have any on hand, put 2/3 cup (67 g) shelled pecans in your food processor with the coconut flour and the salt and pepper and run until it's all finely ground. If you've got pecan meal, just mix it with the other stuff on a plate.

On another plate, mix up the egg with the water.

Throw 2 tablespoons (28 g) of the butter in the skillet to melt.

Dip the chicken in the egg , then in the seasoned pecan meal, then egg, and then pecan meal again, covering both sides. Throw it in the melted butter and cover with a tilted lid. Let it cook a few minutes until crusty on the bottom.

While that's happening, melt 4 tablespoons (55 g) of the butter with the hot sauce—you can do it in a saucepan or nuke it in a microwaveable bowl. This is your Buffalo sauce.

Flip the chicken, throwing the last 2 tablespoons (28 g) of butter in the skillet while you do. Put the tilted lid back on the skillet and cook until crusty on the other side. Plate, top with the Buffalo sauce, and serve with blue cheese dressing for dipping bites in.

Yield: 4 servings, each with 744 calories, 59 grams fat, 44 grams protein, 12 grams carbohydrate, 5 grams dietary fiber, and 7 grams usable carb.

⊕ Shortcut Buffalo Wings

Here's a bonus recipe!

Make your wings according to the method in *The Only 15 Minute Wings I Could Work Out* (See page 100). While they're cooking, make the Buffalo Wing sauce in the recipe above—1/4 cup (55 g) butter melted with 1/4 cup (60 ml) Louisiana-style hot sauce. When the wings are done, toss them with the sauce and serve with blue cheese dressing.

⊕The Only 15-Minute Wings I Could Figure Out

Because I love chicken wings and know that lots of other folks do, too, I tried several ways of cooking them, trying to come up with a way to cook a halfway decent wing within our 15-minute time frame. I'm here to tell you it ain't easy. Frying them took too long and left a big mess. Baked wings were done within 15 minutes if I cranked my oven all the way to 500°F (240°C, or gas mark 9)—but preheating the oven that hot added extra 15 minutes to the process.

Finally I hit on cooking them in my electric tabletop grill, and it worked! My wings were done through, and while they weren't as wonderfully crunchy as oven-baked wings, they were acceptably crisp.

> Chicken wings—as many as will fit in your grill
>> (Mine fits about 8 whole wings.)
>
> Sprinkle-on seasoning of your choice (dry rub barbecue
>> seasoning, jerk seasoning, lemon pepper,
>>
>> Cajun seasoning, Creole seasoning
>>
>> —or just salt and pepper, if you prefer)

Plug your grill in. Do not wait for it to heat up—you need every second of cooking time you can get. Arrange the wings on the grill, pulling them open (extending them at the joints) so they lay as flat as possible on the grill. (Obviously, if you're using cut-up wing "drummettes" this won't be necessary.) Fit as many on the grill as you can. Then sprinkle them with your chosen seasoning and close the grill. Press down gently on the top of the grill, to make sure that the grill is in firm contact with as much of the surface of the wings as possible. Cook for 13 to 15 minutes and serve.

Yield: How many servings you get will depend on the size of your grill. Each wing will have a negligible amount of carbs, no fiber, and 9 grams of protein. (That's for whole wings; figure roughly half that for each "drummette.")

⊕ Lettuce Wraps

These are currently a hot appetizer at Asian restaurants, and they're delicious—but the restaurant version usually contains an unacceptable amount of sugar. Serve these as an appetizer if you like, but I like them as a light supper. Even if you have to make the *Asian Dipping Sauce* (see page 291), too, this comes in under the 15-minute time limit.

1 can (8 ounces, or 225 g) water chestnuts, drained

1 cup (70 g) sliced mushrooms

5 scallions, roots and limp shoot removed, cut into 2 or 3 pieces each

3 tablespoons (45 ml) soy sauce

2 tablespoons (3 g) Splenda

1/2 teaspoon blackstrap molasses

1 1/2 teaspoons minced garlic or 3 cloves of garlic, crushed

1 1/2 teaspoons rice vinegar

3 tablespoons (45 ml) oil

1 pound (455 g) ground chicken

Guar or xanthan

Iceberg or leaf lettuce

Asian Dipping Sauce (see page 291)

Place the water chestnuts, mushrooms, and scallions in your food processor with the S-blade in place. Pulse just enough to chop everything to a medium consistency.

Combine the soy sauce, Splenda, blackstrap molasses, garlic, and rice vinegar. Set aside.

Heat the oil in a wok or large skillet over highest heat. Add the chicken and stir-fry, breaking it up as it cooks. When about half of the pink is gone from the chicken, add the chopped vegetables and stir-fry everything together for a few more minutes. When the chicken is cooked through, stir in the seasoning mixture and let everything cook together for just another minute or so. Thicken the pan juices just a little with guar or xanthan and serve.

To eat this, you wrap spoonfuls of the meat mixture in lettuce leaves, dip the rolls in the *Asian Dipping Sauce*, and then eat them by hand. The tidiest way to do this is to take a whole, firm head of iceberg lettuce and slice a good 2-inch thick (5 cm thick) slab off the side, making lettuce cups—you can do this all over the head, leaving the inside of the head for salad. However, there's no reason not to use leaf lettuce if you prefer it.

Yield: Figure this is 6 servings as an appetizer, each with 10 grams of carbohydrates and 2 grams of fiber, for a total of 8 grams of usable carbs (exclusive of the dipping sauce) and 25 grams of protein, which is a pretty filling appetizer!

Figure this is 4 servings as a main course, each with 15 grams of carbohydrates and 3 grams of fiber, for a total of 12 grams of usable carbs (again, exclusive of the dipping sauce) and 37 grams of protein.

☺ Easy Mexicali Chicken

How simple this is! Yet you know the whole family will like it. Just remember to read the labels to get the lowest-carb salsa.

> 1 1/2 pounds (680 g) boneless, skinless chicken breast
> 2 tablespoons (28 ml) oil
> 4 ounces (115 g) Monterey Jack, pepper Jack, or shredded Mexican cheese blend, as you prefer
> 1/2 cup (130 g) mild, medium, or hot salsa, as you prefer

Pound the chicken breasts to 1/2 inch (1.3 cm) thick and divide into portions, if needed.

Place your large, heavy skillet over medium-high heat, add the oil, and sauté the chicken breasts for about 5 minutes or until the bottom is golden. Turn and sauté for another 3 to 4 minutes. Top the chicken with the cheese, turn the heat down to medium-low, cover the skillet, and let the whole thing cook for another 3 to 4 minutes or until the cheese is melted.

While the cheese is melting, put the salsa in a microwaveable dish and nuke it for a minute at 50 percent power.

Remove the chicken to serving plates, top with the salsa, and serve. You could add a dollop of sour cream if you like or maybe some chopped fresh cilantro, but it's not really necessary.

Yield: 4 or 5 servings. Assuming 4 servings, each will have 2 grams of carbohydrates and 1 gram of fiber, for a total of 1 gram of usable carbs and 45 grams of protein.

⊙ Chicken Liver Sauté

The worst possible thing you can do to liver of any kind is overcook it, which makes chicken livers an ideal candidate for a super-fast gourmet supper. The cauliflower rice is optional with this, but it takes very little extra time, adds only 1 gram of extra carbs to a serving, and makes this seem more like a meal.

1/2 head cauliflower (optional)

8 ounces (225 g) chicken livers

4 ounces (115 g) sliced mushrooms

1/4 medium onion

1 tablespoon (14 g) butter

1/2 teaspoon minced garlic or 1 clove garlic, crushed

1/2 teaspoon ground rosemary*

1/4 cup (60 ml) dry sherry

1/2 teaspoon lemon juice

Salt and pepper

Guar or xanthan

* You can use a teaspoon of dried rosemary needles instead, and it will taste good, but you'll have little tough needles in your food.

If you want cauliflower rice to serve the chicken livers on, make that first. Run the cauliflower through the shredding blade of your food processor, put it in a micro-waveable casserole with a lid, add a couple of tablespoons (28 ml) of water, cover it, and microwave it on High for 7 minutes. If the cauliflower is done cooking before you're quite done with your livers, *remove the lid*. This will let the steam out and stop the cooking. Otherwise you'll get a white mush that bears little resemblance to rice or even cauliflower.

Okay, you're ready to deal with the livers. Cut each liver into 3 or 4 chunks. We're assuming you bought presliced mushrooms, but if you didn't, slice them now. Take the onion quarter, cut it in half again (making two eighths), and then slice it as thin as you can.

Melt the butter in a large, heavy skillet over medium-high heat. Add the livers, mushrooms, onions, and garlic and stir-fry until the mushrooms are starting to change color and most of the pink is gone from the livers. Add the rosemary, sherry, lemon juice, and a little salt and pepper and let it all simmer for just 1 to 2 minutes. Thicken the pan liquid slightly with guar or xanthan and serve, with or without cauliflower rice.

Yield: 2 servings. Without the cauliflower rice, each serving will have 8 grams of carbohydrates and 1 gram of fiber, for a total of 7 grams of usable carbs and 22 grams of protein.

If you serve it with the cauliflower rice, each serving will have 10 grams of carbohydrates and 2 grams of fiber, for a total of 8 grams of usable carbs and 22 grams of protein.

⏲ Lemon~Glazed Turkey Cutlets

Turkey cutlets—slices of turkey breast less than 1/4 inch (6 mm) thick—are good for cooks in a hurry because they take almost no time to cook through. They're pretty bland by themselves, however, and can easily turn dry and tough. But they take beautifully to this tart-sweet lemon glaze.

> 3 turkey cutlets, about 4 ounces (115 g) each
>
> 1 tablespoon (15 ml) olive oil
>
> 1 tablespoon (15 ml) lemon juice
>
> 1 tablespoon (15 ml) dry sherry
>
> 2 teaspoons Splenda
>
> 1/2 teaspoon soy sauce
>
> Guar or xanthan
>
> 3 scallions, finely sliced

In a large, heavy skillet over medium heat, brown the cutlets in the oil. While that's happening, mix together the lemon juice, sherry, Splenda, soy sauce, and just a sprinkle of guar or xanthan to thicken the mixture. When the cutlets have just a touch of golden color on each side, pour the lemon juice mixture into the skillet and turn the cutlets over once to coat both sides. Turn the burner to medium-low, cover, and let the cutlets simmer for just a few more minutes until the sauce reduces a little.

Serve with any glaze left in the pan scraped over the cutlets and a sliced scallion scattered over each.

Yield: 2 or 3 servings. Assuming 2 servings, each will have 4 grams of carbohydrates and 1 gram of fiber, for a total of 3 grams of usable carbs and 37 grams of protein.

⊕ Mustard-Pecan Turkey Cutlets

Of all the things I've tried with turkey cutlets, this is my husband's favorite. The mustard-mayo coating keeps these from getting dry.

> 1/2 cup (50 g) shelled pecans
>
> 1 tablespoon (11 g) spicy brown or Dijon mustard
>
> 3 tablespoons (42 g) mayonnaise
>
> 3 turkey breast cutlets, about 4 ounces (115 g) each
>
> 1 1/2 tablespoons (21 g) butter

Place the pecans in your food processor with the S-blade in place and pulse until they're ground medium-fine. (Alternately, you could buy the pecans already ground.)

Mix together the mustard and mayonnaise, blending well.

Lay the turkey cutlets on a plate and spread half of the mustard and mayonnaise mixture on one side. Sprinkle half of the ground pecans over the mustard and mayonnaise and press lightly with the back of a spoon to help them stick.

Spray a large, heavy skillet with nonstick cooking spray. Place over medium-high heat. Melt the butter and add the cutlets, pecan side down. Sauté for about 4 minutes. With the cutlets still in the pan, spread the remaining mustard-mayo mixture on the uncoated sides and sprinkle the rest of the pecans over that, once again pressing them in a bit with the back of a spoon. Flip the cutlets carefully, doing your best not to dislodge the crust. Sauté for another 5 minutes and serve. Scrape any yummy toasted pecans that are stuck to the skillet over the cutlets before serving.

Yield: 2 or 3 servings. Assuming 2 servings, each will have 4 grams of carbohydrates and 2 grams of fiber, for a total of 2 grams of usable carbs and 39 grams of protein.

chapter five

15~Minute
Fish and Seafood

If you're trying to eat low-carb and to be as healthy as possible on a tight schedule, you just can't do any better than fish. Of course we know fish is wonderful for us, but it's also to our advantage that it's hard to find a fish recipe that calls for more than 15 minutes' cooking time!

Indeed, the only thing I can think of to say against fish is that it is often expensive. Around here, the fish we eat most often are catfish, tilapia, and whiting, for the simple reason that they're the fish that are cheapest, at least here in the Midwest.

However, fish are frequently interchangeable in recipes, so if you prefer sole, orange roughy, cod, flounder, or what-have-you, don't hesitate to try them. There's no reason why they shouldn't work out fine, with a little adjustment of time for thicker or thinner fillets.

⊕ Shrimp Stewed in Curry Butter

Don't bother with napkins, just put the roll of paper towels on the table
—this is messy! It's delicious, though.

> 6 tablespoons (85 g) butter
>
> 2 teaspoons curry powder
>
> 1 teaspoon minced garlic or 2 cloves garlic, crushed
>
> 24 large, raw, "easy peel" shrimp

Melt the butter in a large, heavy skillet over lowest heat. Stir in the curry powder
and garlic and then add the shrimp in a single layer. Cook for 3 to 5 minutes per side
or until the shrimp are pink right through. Transfer to serving plates and scrape the
extra curry butter over them.

Yield: 2 servings, each with 2 grams of carbohydrates, 1 gram of fiber (if you lick
up every last drop of the curry-garlic butter), for a total of a bit less than 1 gram
of usable carbs per serving and 15 grams of protein.

⊕ Saigon Shrimp

There are vietnamese style—hot and a little sweet.

> Scant 1/2 teaspoon salt
>
> Scant 1/2 teaspoon pepper
>
> 1 1/2 teaspoons Splenda
>
> 3 scallions
>
> 4 tablespoons (60 ml) peanut or canola oil
>
> 1 pound (455 g) large shrimp, shelled and deveined
>
> 1 1/2 teaspoons chili garlic paste
>
> 2 teaspoons minced garlic

Mix together the salt, pepper, and Splenda in a small dish or cup. Slice the
scallions thinly and set them aside. Gather all the ingredients except the scallions
together—the actual cooking of this dish is lightning fast!

In a wok or heavy skillet over highest heat, heat the oil. Add the shrimp and stir-fry
for 2 to 3 minutes or until they're about two-thirds pink. Add the chili garlic paste

and garlic and keep stir-frying. When the shrimp are pink all over and all the way through, sprinkle the salt, pepper, and Splenda mixture over them and stir for just another 10 seconds or so. Turn off the heat and divide the shrimp between 3 serving plates. Top each serving with a scattering of sliced scallion and serve.

Yield: 3 servings, each with 2 grams of carbohydrates and 1 gram of fiber, for a total of 1 gram of usable carbs and 25 grams of protein.

✳ This dish comes in at a low 288 calories a serving.

⊕ Basil-Lime Shrimp

 1/2 cup (120 ml) lime juice

 1/2 cup (120 ml) olive oil

 1/4 cup (10 g) fresh basil—Just compact sprigs into your measuring cup.

 4 teaspoons (16 g) brown mustard

 1/4 teaspoon Splenda

 4 scallions—thinly sliced, including the crisp part of the green

 1/2 pound (225 g) shrimp

Put everything from the lime juice through the Splenda in your blender and run it just for a second or two. Pour the mixture into a big nonreactive pan and place over medium heat. Bring to a simmer, turn the heat down to keep it just simmering, and let it cook until it's reduced by about half. While that's happening, slice your scallions.

When the lime juice mixture is reduced, lay the shrimp in it, in one layer if possible. (If not, you'll have to stir them around some.) Let them poach for about two minutes and then flip and give them another couple of minutes, just until they're firm and pink. Serve drizzled with the sauce, with the sliced scallion sprinkled over the top.

Yield: 4 servings, each with 438 calories, 30 grams fat, 35 grams protein, 6 grams carbohydrate, 1 gram dietary fiber, and 5 grams usable carb.

Note: The carb count on this only holds if you consume all of the sauce. If you leave some on your plate, you leave a few carbs behind, too, but get the benefit of the flavor.

⊕ Shrimp in Brandy Cream

Wow—this is sheer elegance. And it's done in a flash!

> 1 pound (455 g) shrimp, shelled and deveined
>
> 4 tablespoons (55 g) butter
>
> 1/3 cup (80 ml) brandy
>
> 3/4 cup (175 ml) heavy cream
>
> Guar or xanthan (optional)

Sauté the shrimp in the butter over medium-high heat until cooked through—4 to 5 minutes. Add the brandy, turn up the heat, and let it boil hard for a minute or so to reduce. Stir in the cream and heat through. Thicken the sauce a bit with guar or xanthan if you like and then serve.

Yield: 3 or 4 servings. Assuming 3 servings, each will have 2 grams of carbohydrates, no fiber, and 26 grams of protein.

⊕ Shrimp in Curried Coconut Milk

Coconut is emerging as a true super-food, and it certainly gives this dish a rich, exotic flavor. This is stew-like; serve it in bowls.

1/2 onion

1/2 green pepper

2 tablespoons (28 ml) coconut oil

2 teaspoons cumin

2 teaspoons curry powder

1 1/2 teaspoons ground coriander

1 1/2 teaspoons chopped garlic

1 cup (235 ml) unsweetened coconut milk

1/2 teaspoon salt or Vege-Sal

1/4 teaspoon chili garlic paste

3 cups (384) frozen cooked salad shrimp, thawed

Throw your onion and green pepper in the food processor and pulse until they're chopped fine. In a heavy-bottomed skillet, start them sautéing in the coconut oil over medium heat.

When the onion and pepper are starting to soften, throw in the spices. Sauté another few minutes, add the garlic, and give it just another minute.

Add the coconut milk and stir the whole thing up. Stir in the salt and chili garlic paste, too.

Now add the thawed, drained shrimp, stir it in, and turn the burner up a little. Simmer for a minute or two, thickening with a little guar, xanthan, or glucomannan if you think it needs it. Then serve—with spoons, to get all of the sauce!

Yield: 3 servings, each with 235 calories, 11 grams fat, 28 grams protein, 6 grams carbohydrate, 1 gram dietary fiber, and 5 grams usable carb.

⊕ Salmon in Ginger Cream

This has all the goodness of salmon in an elegant sauce.

> 2 tablespoons (28 g) butter
>
> 2 pieces salmon fillet, 6 ounces (170 g) each, skin still attached
>
> 1 teaspoon minced garlic or 2 cloves garlic, crushed
>
> 2 scallions, finely minced
>
> 2 tablespoons (2 g) chopped cilantro
>
> 4 tablespoons (60 ml) dry white wine
>
> 2 tablespoons (16 g) grated gingerroot
>
> 4 tablespoons (60 g) sour cream
>
> Salt and pepper

Melt the butter in a heavy skillet over medium-low heat and start sautéing the salmon in it—you want to sauté it for about 4 minutes per side.

While the fish is sautéing, crush the garlic, mince the scallions, and chop the cilantro.

When both sides of the salmon have sautéed for 4 minutes, add the wine to the skillet, cover, and let the fish cook an additional 2 minutes or so until done through. Remove the fish to serving plates.

Add the garlic, scallions, cilantro, and ginger to the wine and butter in the skillet, turn the burner up to medium-high, and let them cook for a minute or two. Add the sour cream, stir to blend, and salt and pepper to taste. Spoon the sauce over the fish and serve.

Yield: 2 servings, each with 5 grams of carbohydrates and 1 gram of fiber, for a total of 4 grams of usable carbs and 36 grams of protein

✽ This dish also has lots of EPA—the good fat that makes salmon so heart-healthy!

⊕ Buttered Salmon with Creole Seasonings

12 ounces (340 g) salmon fillet, in two or three pieces

1 teaspoon purchased Creole seasoning

1/4 teaspoon dried thyme

4 tablespoons (55 g) butter

1 teaspoon minced garlic or 2 cloves garlic, minced

Sprinkle the skinless side of the salmon evenly with the Creole seasoning and thyme. Melt the butter in a heavy skillet over medium-low heat and add the salmon, skin side down. Cook 4 to 5 minutes per side, turning carefully. Remove to serving plates, skin side down, and stir the garlic into the butter remaining in the pan. Cook for just a minute, then scrape all the garlic butter over the salmon, and serve.

Yield: 2 or 3 servings. Assuming 2 servings, each will have 2 grams of carbohydrates and a trace of fiber, for a total of 2 grams of usable carbs and 35 grams of protein.

⊕ Glazed, Grilled Salmon

Of all the ways I've cooked salmon, this drew the most praise.

> 2 tablespoons (3 g) Splenda
>
> 1 1/2 teaspoons dry mustard
>
> 1 tablespoon (15 ml) soy sauce
>
> 1 1/2 teaspoons rice vinegar
>
> 1/4 teaspoon blackstrap molasses, or the darkest molasses you can find
>
> 12 ounces (340 g) salmon fillet, cut into 2 or 3 serving-size pieces

Mix together the Splenda, mustard, soy sauce, vinegar, and molasses in a small dish. Spoon out 1 tablespoon (15 g) of this mixture and set it aside in a separate dish.

Place the salmon fillets on a plate and pour the larger quantity of the soy sauce mixture over it, turning each fillet so that both sides come in contact with the seasonings. Let the fish sit for a few minutes—just 2 or 3—with the skinless side down in the seasonings.

Now, you get to choose how you want to cook the salmon. I do mine on a stove top grill, but you can broil it, do it in a heavy skillet sprayed with nonstick cooking spray, cook it on your electric tabletop grill, or even do it on your outdoor grill. However you cook it, it will need about 5 minutes per side (or just 5 minutes total, in an electric grill). If you choose a method that requires you to turn the salmon, turn carefully! Baste once, when turning, with the soy sauce mixture you reserved. (Don't do it after that—you want the heat to kill any raw fish germs!)

When the salmon is cooked through, remove it to serving plates and drizzle the reserved seasoning mixture over each piece before serving.

Yield: This makes 2 generous servings or 3 smaller ones. Assuming 2 servings, each will have 3 grams of carbohydrates, a trace of fiber, and 35 grams of protein.

⊕ Peach Salmon

This makes a fruity-good summer supper.

> 24 ounces (680 g) salmon fillet in four servings
>
> 3 tablespoons (42 g) butter
>
> 2 fresh peaches
>
> 1/4 onion
>
> 1 teaspoon chopped garlic
>
> 1 1/2 teaspoons curry powder
>
> 2 tablespoons (28 ml) lemon juice
>
> 1/4 cup (6 g) Splenda or its equivalent in sweetness
>
> salt and pepper

Start the salmon sautéing in the butter over medium heat and cover it with a tilted lid.

Peel your peaches, halve, and remove the pits. Throw the peaches, onion, garlic, and curry powder in your food processor and pulse until the peach is chopped medium-fine. Go flip your salmon.

Mix together the lemon juice and Splenda. When your salmon is done through, plate it. Pour the lemon juice mixture in the skillet and stir it around, scraping up the yummy brown bits. Add the peach mixture and cook for just a minute or two, stirring. Salt and pepper to taste and then spoon over the salmon and serve.

Yield: 4 servings, each with 309 calories, 15 grams fat, 35 grams protein, 9 grams carbohydrate, 1 gram dietary fiber, and 8 grams usable carb.

⊕ Salmon in Citrus Vinaigrette

My husband said this was perhaps the best salmon dish he'd ever had.

> 1 tablespoon (15 ml) coconut oil
>
> 24 ounces (680 g) salmon fillet in 4 servings
>
> 1/2 cup (120 ml) vinaigrette (I used Paul Newman's light red wine vinegar and olive oil.)
>
> 1/2 cup (120 ml) lemon juice
>
> 2 1/2 tablespoons (4 g) Splenda, or the equivalent in liquid Splenda
>
> 1/4 teaspoon orange extract
>
> 1 teaspoon brown mustard
>
> 1 teaspoon chili powder
>
> 2 tablespoons (28 ml) lime juice

Spray a big skillet with nonstick cooking spray and put it over medium heat. Throw in the coconut oil and when it's melted, slosh it around and then add the salmon.

While the salmon is getting a little touch of gold, throw everything else in the blender and run the thing.

Okay, go back and flip your salmon. Let it get a little gold on the other side, too.

Now add the vinaigrette mixture and turn the burner up to medium-high. Let the whole thing cook another five minutes or until the salmon is done through.

Plate the salmon and turn up the burner. Boil the vinaigrette hard until it's reduced and starting to get a little syrupy. Pour over the salmon and serve.

Yield: 4 servings, each with 384 calories, 25 grams fat, 34 grams protein, 5 grams carbohydrate, trace dietary fiber, and 5 grams usable carb.

⊕ Skillet Barbecued Salmon

Don't panic at this list of ingredients; this really is quick and easy.

1/4 cup (115 g) bacon grease

24 ounces (680 g) salmon fillets, 1-inch (2.5 cm) thick and cut into four
servings

2 tablespoons (28 ml) pineapple juice, or sugar-free pineapple syrup (DaVinci
makes this.)

1/4 cup (60 ml) soy sauce

1 1/3 tablespoons (20 ml) rice vinegar

1 1/3 tablespoons (20 ml) lemon juice

2 teaspoons olive oil

1/2 cup (12 g) Splenda

1/8 cup erythritol

1/3 teaspoon molasses

1/2 teaspoon pepper

1/3 teaspoon cayenne

1/3 teaspoon paprika

1/8 teaspoon garlic

Put your big, heavy skillet over medium-high heat and throw in the bacon grease.
When it's hot, add the fillets. Let them sizzle there while you mix together everything else.

Flip your fillets after 4 to 5 minutes and let them get golden on the other side, too.

Now pour in the sauce and flip the fillets again to coat. Let them simmer in the
sauce until they're done through. Then plate the fillets and turn up the burner. Boil
the sauce until it's syrupy, pour over the fillets, and serve.

Yield: 4 servings, each with 366 calories, 21 grams fat, 35 grams protein, 7 grams
carbohydrate, trace dietary fiber, and 7 grams usable carb.

⊕ Whiting with Mexican Flavors

I made this for lunch when a friend of my husband's was visiting town, and
we all agreed it was one of the best things I've ever made.

> 4 whiting fillets
>
> 2 tablespoons (28 ml) lime juice
>
> 3/4 teaspoon chili powder
>
> 2 tablespoons (28 ml) oil
>
> 1 medium onion
>
> 2 tablespoons (28 ml) orange juice
>
> 1/2 teaspoon Splenda
>
> 1/4 teaspoon ground cumin
>
> 1/4 teaspoon dried oregano
>
> 1 tablespoon (15 ml) white wine vinegar
>
> 1/2 teaspoon hot sauce
>
> Salt and pepper

Lay the whiting fillets on a plate and sprinkle with 1 tablespoon (15 ml) of lime juice,
turning to coat. Sprinkle the skinless sides of the fillets with chili powder.

Heat the oil in a heavy skillet over medium heat. Add the whiting fillets. Sauté for
about 4 minutes per side, turning carefully, or until cooked through. Remove to a
serving plate and keep warm.

Add the onions to the skillet and turn the heat up to medium-high. Sauté the
onions for a couple of minutes until they begin to go limp. Stir in the orange juice,
Splenda, cumin, oregano, vinegar, and hot sauce. Cook them all together for a
minute or two. Salt and pepper to taste. Spoon the onions over the fish and serve.

Yield: 4 servings, each with 5 grams of carbohydrates and 1 gram of fiber,
for a total of 4 grams of usable carbs and 17 grams of protein.

✳ Each serving has only 162 calories!

☺Coconut Crusted Flounder with Browned Butter and Lime

1/2 cup (63 g) coconut flour

salt and pepper or Vege-Sal

3 eggs

1 1/2 pounds (680 g) flounder fillet

1 stick butter, divided

1 lime

4 tablespoons (16 g) minced fresh parsley

Give your big, heavy skillet a squirt of nonstick cooking spray and set it to heating over a medium burner.

On a plate, mix the coconut flour with the salt and pepper—maybe 1/4 teaspoon each.

On another plate with a rim, beat up the eggs with a tablespoon (15 ml) of water.

Throw half the butter in the skillet and let it melt.

Dip each fillet in the egg, then in the coconut flour, then egg, then flour, twice, on both sides. Throw them in the hot butter!

Give your fish about 4 to 5 minutes per side until nice and crusty brown. Add a little more butter if you need to when you turn the fish. When it's brown on both sides, plate it.

Now throw the rest of the butter in the hot skillet and let it melt and then brown. Pour the browned butter over the flounder fillets. Top with parsley and serve with a wedge of lime.

Yield: 4 servings, each with 540 calories, 32 grams fat, 41 grams protein, 24 grams carbohydrate, 13 grams dietary fiber, and 11 grams usable carb.

☉ Transcendent Flounder

This recipe is so-called because my husband took one bite and said, "That's transcendent!"

1/4 cup (55 g) butter

2 pounds (900 g) flounder fillets, cut into four pieces

2 lemons

1/3 cup (75 g) mayonnaise

1/3 cup (33 g) grated Parmesan cheese

4 scallions

Turn on your broiler and arrange a rack about 4 inches (10 cm) beneath.

Put the butter in a custard cup or glass measuring cup and microwave it for a minute to melt.

Lay a piece of foil over your broiler pan and spray it with nonstick cooking spray. Cup the edges a little. Now lay out the flounder fillets. Pour the butter evenly over the fillets and use a brush or the back of a spoon to make sure they're coated all over. Halve the lemons, pick out the seeds, and squeeze the juice over the fish.

Slide the fish under the broiler. While it's cooking, measure and mix together the mayo and Parmesan.

By now your fillets should be getting close to done; it doesn't take long. If they're cooking unevenly, turn the pan and let them cook another minute.

When the flounder is getting opaque and flaky, spread the mayonnaise mixture evenly over them and slide them back under the broiler.

Slice up your scallions. Then check your fish—again, if the topping is browning unevenly, turn the pan to even it out and give it another minute or two. When the topping is evenly golden, plate the fish, scatter sliced scallion over each serving, and eat.

Yield: 4 servings, each with 481 calories, 32 grams fat, 46 grams protein, 4 grams carbohydrate, 1 gram dietary fiber, and 3 grams usable carb.

◷ Chinese Steamed Fish

I made this with tilapia, and while it was quite tasty, it was also fragile. If you're willing to pay the difference for a firmer fish like orange roughy or cod, it will be easier to handle.

12 ounces (340 g) fish fillets

2 tablespoons (28 ml) dry sherry

1 tablespoon (15 ml) soy sauce

2 teaspoons grated gingerroot

1/2 teaspoon minced garlic or 1 clove garlic, crushed

1 1/2 teaspoons toasted sesame oil

1 or 2 scallions, minced (optional)

Lay the fish fillets on a piece of heavy-duty aluminum foil and turn the edges up to form a lip.

Mix together the sherry, soy sauce, gingerroot, garlic, and sesame oil.

Fit a rack—a cake-cooling rack works nicely—into a large skillet. Pour about 1/4 inch (6 mm) of water in the bottom of the skillet and turn the heat to high. Place the foil with the fish on it on the rack. Carefully pour the sherry mixture over the fish. Cover the pan tightly.

Cook for 5 to 7 minutes or until the fish flakes easily. Serve with minced scallions as a garnish, if desired.

Yield: 2 servings, each with 2 grams of carbohydrates, no fiber, and 31 grams of protein.

✴ Each serving has only 195 calories!

Three Ridiculously Easy Things To Do with Catfish

(Plus One That's Only a Tiny Bit More Complicated)

You'll notice a certain similarity between these three recipes, but they all taste quite different—and quite good! Personally, I think coleslaw (with sugar-free dressing, of course) would make an ideal side dish with any of these recipes, but then again, I'm inordinately fond of coleslaw. Despite the butter, all three of these recipes come in at under 300 calories per serving, as well as being very low carb.

⊕ Lemon-Pepper Catfish

> 1 pound (455 g) catfish fillets
>
> Lemon pepper
>
> 3 to 4 tablespoons (42 to 55 g) butter

Sprinkle both sides of the catfish fillets liberally with lemon pepper and let them sit for 5 minutes. Melt the butter over medium heat in a heavy skillet. Add the catfish, sauté for about 5 minutes per side or until cooked through, and then serve.

Yield: 3 servings, each with 1 gram of carbohydrates, a trace of fiber, and 25 grams of protein.

⊕ Old Bay Catfish

> 1 pound (455 g) catfish fillets
>
> Old Bay Seasoning*
>
> 3 to 4 tablespoons (42 to 55 g) butter

* This is a widely available sprinkle-on seasoning; look for it in your grocery store.

Sprinkle both sides of the catfish fillets liberally with Old Bay Seasoning and let them sit for 5 minutes. Melt the butter over medium heat in a heavy skillet. Add the catfish, sauté for about 5 minutes per side or until cooked through, and then serve.

Yield: 3 servings, each with just a trace of carbohydrates, no fiber, and 25 grams of protein.

⊕ Creole Catfish

> 1 pound (455 g) catfish fillets
> Creole seasoning
> 3 to 4 tablespoons (42 to 55 g) butter

Sprinkle both sides of the catfish fillets liberally with Creole seasoning and let them sit for 5 minutes. Melt the butter over medium heat in a heavy skillet. Add the catfish, sauté for about 5 minutes per side or until cooked through, and then serve.

Yield: 3 servings, each with 2 grams of carbohydrates, a trace of fiber, and 25 grams of protein.

⊕ Crunchy Creole Catfish

That's nice alliteration, huh? If you have some crushed BBQ pork rinds on hand, this is a tasty elaboration on the previous catfish recipe.

> 1 pound (455 g) catfish fillets
> Creole seasoning
> 1/3 cup (80 g) crushed barbeque-flavor pork rinds
> 3 tablespoons (42 g) butter

Sprinkle the catfish fillets liberally on both sides with Creole seasoning. Spread the pork rind crumbs on a plate and dip both sides of each fillet in the crumbs to coat. Melt the butter in a heavy skillet over medium heat and sauté the fillets for 4 to 5 minutes per side or until cooked through and crispy.

Yield: 2-3 servings, each with 2 grams of carbohydrates, a trace of fiber and 46 grams of protein.

⏲ Oysters en Brochette

Oysters are an oddity in the world of animal protein, in that they actually contain a few carbs of their own. Still, they're quite nutritious (loaded with zinc) and many people love them. This makes an elegant appetizer or a very light supper.

> 6 slices bacon
>
> 24 mushrooms
>
> 16 large oysters
>
> Butter (optional)
>
> Lemon wedges (optional)

You'll either need metal skewers for this or you'll need to think far enough ahead to put 6 bamboo skewers in water to soak for a few hours before you begin cooking.

Either way, simply skewer a slice of bacon near the end and then skewer a mushroom. Fold the strip of bacon back over, skewering it again, then add an oyster, and fold and skewer the bacon again—you're weaving the bacon in and out of the alternating mushrooms and oysters, see?

Lay the skewers on a broiler pan and broil them close to the heat with the broiler on Low for about 10 minutes. Turn once or twice until the oysters are done and the bacon's getting crisp. You can baste these with butter while they're broiling if you like, but it's not strictly necessary. Serve one skewer per customer as a first course, with lemon wedges if you like.

Yield: 3 servings, each with 8 grams of carbohydrates and 2 grams of fiber, for a total of 6 grams of usable carbs and 10 grams of protein.

Two Variations: My husband, who refers to mushrooms as "slime," likes these without the mushrooms. This cuts the carb count down to just 2 grams per serving.

If you'd like to impress the guests at your next party, you can cut strips of bacon in half and wrap each half-strip around an oyster, piercing with a toothpick to hold. Broil as above until the bacon gets crispy and serve hot. These are called Angels on Horseback—I have no idea why—and they're a classic hot hors d'oeuvre. These will have just a trace of carbohydrates per piece.

☺White Clam and Bacon Pizza or Omelet Filling

My husband really loved his White Clam and Bacon Omelet!

4 slices bacon

1 tablespoon bacon grease (15 g) or olive oil (15 ml)

3 tablespoons (30 g) minced onion

1 teaspoon chopped garlic

1 can (6 ½ ounces, or 180 g) minced clams

1 teaspoon Italian seasoning

¼ cup (15 g) chopped fresh parsley

½ cup (58 g) 6 cheese Italian shredded cheese blend or shredded mozzarella

Lay your bacon on a microwave bacon rack or in a Pyrex pie plate and give it 4 to 6 minutes on high in the microwave.

Over medium heat, melt the bacon grease (this would be from bacon you cooked some other time—you are keeping your bacon grease to cook with, right? If you don't have bacon grease, use olive oil) in a medium-sized skillet and start sautéing the onion. While that's happening, open and drain the clams and chop your parsley.

When the onion's translucent, add the garlic, drained clams, and Italian seasoning and keep cooking until most of the residual liquid cooks away. Stir in the parsley and give it just another minute.

Okay, now you have a choice: You can make omelets according to *Dana's Easy Omelet Method*, putting ¼ cup (30 g) of cheese in first, then the clam mixture, and topping with two strips of crumbled bacon. Or you can make tortilla pizzas, layering the same way, but heating the oven might run you past 15 minutes.

Yield: 2 servings, each with 471 calories, 29 grams fat, 43 grams protein, 9 grams carbohydrate, 1 gram dietary fiber, and 8 grams usable carb.

⊕ Microwaved Fish and Asparagus with Tarragon Mustard Sauce

Microwaving is a great way to cook vegetables and a great way to cook fish—so it's a natural way to cook combinations of the two.

    10 asparagus spears

    2 tablespoons (30 g) sour cream

    1 tablespoon (14 g) mayonnaise

    1/4 teaspoon dried tarragon

    1/2 teaspoon Dijon or spicy brown mustard

    12 ounces (340 g) fish fillets—whiting, tilapia, sole, flounder,
        or any other mild white fish

Snap the bottoms off the asparagus spears where they break naturally. Place the asparagus in a large glass pie plate, add 1 tablespoon (15 ml) of water, and cover by placing a plate on top. Microwave on High for 3 minutes.

While the asparagus is microwaving, stir together the sour cream, mayonnaise, tarragon, and mustard.

Remove the asparagus from the microwave, take it out of the pie plate, and set it aside. Drain the water out of the pie plate. Place the fish fillets in the pie plate and spread 2 tablespoons (28 g) of the sour cream mixture over them. Re-cover the pie plate and microwave the fish for 3 to 4 minutes on High. Open the microwave, remove the plate from the top of the pie plate, and arrange the asparagus on top of the fish. Re-cover the pie plate and cook for another 1 to 2 minutes on High.

Remove the pie plate from the microwave and take the plate off. Place the fish and asparagus on serving plates. Scrape any sauce that's cooked into the pie plate over the fish and asparagus. Top each serving with the reserved sauce and serve.

Yield: 2 servings, each with 4 grams of carbohydrates and 2 grams of fiber, for a total of 2 grams of usable carbs and 33 grams of protein.

✷ This dish also packs in 949 milligrams of potassium!

⊕ California Tuna Fritters

This makes a quick and different supper out of simple canned tuna. You can make this into a few big tuna burgers, if you prefer, and cut a few minutes off the cooking time, but we really like these as little fritters.

1 stalk celery

6 scallions

1/2 green pepper

2 tablespoons (8 g) chopped fresh parsley

1 egg

1 tablespoon (11 g) spicy brown mustard or Dijon mustard

12 ounces (340 g) canned water-pack tuna, drained

1/3 cup (53 g) rice protein powder

4 to 5 tablespoons (55 to 70 g) butter

Plunk the celery, scallions, pepper, parsley, egg, and mustard in a food processor with the S-blade in place and pulse until the vegetables are chopped to a medium-fine consistency. Add the tuna and rice protein and pulse to mix.

Spray a large, heavy skillet with nonstick cooking spray and place over medium-high heat. Melt 2 to 3 tablespoons (28 to 42 g) of butter in it and drop in the tuna mixture by the tablespoonful. Fry until brown, turn, and brown other side. It takes two batches to cook all of this mixture in my skillet; add the rest of the butter when you make the second batch. Serve with *Easy Remoulade Sauce* (see page 293), which takes all of 2 or 3 minutes to make.

Yield: 4 or 5 servings. Assuming 5 servings, and not including the *Easy Remoulade Sauce*, each will have 5 grams of carbohydrates and 1 gram of fiber, for a total of 4 grams of usable carbs and 32 grams of protein.

⊙ Ginger Mustard Fish

> 4 fish fillets, about 6 ounces (170 g) each—tilapia, cod,
>
>   orange roughy, what ever have you
>
> 4 tablespoons (55 g) butter
>
> 2 teaspoons minced garlic or 4 cloves garlic, crushed
>
> 2 teaspoons grated gingerroot
>
> 2 teaspoons spicy brown or Dijon mustard
>
> 1 tablespoon (15 ml) water

In a large, heavy skillet, start sautéing the fish in the butter over medium-low heat; 4 to 5 minutes per side should be plenty. Remove the fish to a plate.

Add the garlic, gingerroot, mustard, and water to the skillet and stir everything together well. Put the fish back in, turning it over once, carefully, to make sure both sides get acquainted with the sauce. Let it cook for another minute or so and then serve. Scrape the sauce out of the skillet over the fish.

Yield: 4 servings, each with 1 gram of carbohydrates, a trace of fiber, and 31 grams of protein.

⊕ Swordfish Veracruz

This is so simple and quick—yet it's the sort of thing you'd pay big bucks for at a fancy restaurant. Salsa verde is a green salsa made from tomatillos. Look for it in the Mexican or International section of your grocery store.

> 24 ounces (680 g) swordfish steaks
>
> 1/2 cup (120 ml) ruby red grapefruit juice—I like to use fresh-squeezed.
>
> 1/2 teaspoon ground cumin
>
> 1 tablespoon oil
>
> 1/4 cup (65 g) salsa verde

Cut the swordfish into 4 servings and place on a plate with a rim. Mix together the grapefruit juice and the cumin and pour it over the steaks, turning them to coat both sides. Let the swordfish steaks sit in the grapefruit juice for 5 minutes or so.

Spray a large, heavy skillet with nonstick cooking spray and place over medium heat. When the skillet is hot, add the oil and then the fish. Sauté for 4 minutes per side. Then pour in the grapefruit juice from the plate and let the fish cook in it for another minute or two, turning once.

Place the fish on serving plates, top each serving with a tablespoon of salsa verde, and serve.

Yield: 4 servings, each with 4 grams of carbohydrates, a trace of fiber, and 34 grams of protein.

Variation: You can expand this recipe a bit by serving the fish on a bed of avocado slices—split one avocado between the 4 servings—and sprinkling chopped fresh cilantro on top. This will take you up to 8 grams of carbohydrates per serving and 2 grams of fiber, for a total of 6 grams of usable carbs.

⊕ Truite au Bleu

This is more a method of preparation than a recipe, and it's a true classic. Expand or contract this recipe at will to serve however many diners you have.

Water

Cider vinegar

Bay leaves

Peppercorns or coarse cracked pepper

Salt or Vege-Sal

Trout, cleaned and beheaded, but with the skin still on—about 10 ounces (280 g) per serving as a main course, or 5 or 6 ounces (140 to 170 g) per serving as a first course

Butter

You'll need a pan big enough for the trout to lie flat—I generally do just one big trout, weighing about a pound (455 g), and the only pan I have where it can lie flat is my big soup kettle. Use what you have, but it should be a pan that won't react with acid—stainless steel, enamelware, anodized aluminum, or stove-top glassware.

Next, you make up a solution of water and vinegar, just enough to completely cover the trout. The proportions you want are roughly 3 or 4 parts water to 1 part vinegar. I find that 1 1/2 quarts (1.4 L) of water and 1 1/2 cups (355 ml) of vinegar are about right for my pan. Pour this solution in your pan and turn the burner to high. Stir in 1 or 2 bay leaves, 1/2 tablespoon of pepper per quart (950 ml), and 1 teaspoon of salt or Vege-Sal per quart (950 ml). Bring this mixture to a simmer.

Simply lower the trout into the simmering solution, turn the burner to medium-low, and let the fish simmer for about 5 minutes. Lift the fish carefully out of the simmering solution and serve with a pitcher of melted butter to pour over the fish.

Yield: Servings will depend on how many fish you cook, of course. The fish itself is carb-free, and of course, most of the poaching solution is discarded—you can figure on no more than a gram of carbohydrates per serving, no fiber, and 59 grams of protein in a 10-ounce (280 g) trout.

⊕ Mock Lobster

Monkfish has long been known as "poor man's lobster," so I decided to play up the similarity. Your microwave is great for cooking fish, and as for quick, let's face it—if this dish cooked any faster, you'd go back in time. Feel free to double or triple this. You'll just need to use a bigger plate (a glass pie plate will work beautifully) and add just a minute or two extra cooking time.

> 1 1/2 tablespoons (21 g) butter
> 6 ounces (170 g) monkfish fillet
> Lemon wedges

Put the butter on a microwaveable plate. Nuke it for 30 seconds at 70 percent power or until melted.

Place the monkfish in the butter and turn it over to coat both sides. Cover the fish with microwave-safe plastic wrap. Nuke for 1 1/2 minutes at 50 percent power. Uncover the fish, turn it over, and recover with the plastic wrap. Nuke for 30 seconds more at 50 percent power. Let it stand for a minute (or if you're making another serving, a minute or two more), remove the plastic wrap, and check for doneness. If necessary, re-cover and give it another 30 seconds or so and then serve with lemon wedges.

Yield: 1 serving, with only a trace of carbohydrates, no fiber, and 25 grams of protein.

⊕ Mock Lobster with Garlic

You'll notice a certain similarity to the previous recipe, but garlic changes the whole flavor.

> 1 1/2 tablespoons (21 g) butter
>
> 1/2 teaspoon minced garlic or 1 clove garlic, crushed
>
> 6 ounces (170 g) monkfish fillet

Put the butter on a microwaveable plate. Nuke it for 30 seconds at 70 percent power or until melted. Stir the garlic into the butter.

Place the monkfish in the butter and turn it over to coat both sides. Cover the fish with microwave-safe plastic wrap. Nuke for 1 1/2 minutes at 50 percent power. Uncover the fish, turn it over, and recover with the plastic wrap. Nuke for 30 seconds more at 50 percent power. Let it stand for a minute (or if you're making another serving, a minute or two more), remove the plastic wrap and check for doneness. If necessary, re-cover and give it another 30 seconds or so and then serve.

Yield: 1 serving, with only a trace of carbohydrates, no fiber, and 25 grams of protein.

⊕ Sea Bass with Tapenade Cream Sauce

Here's another one of those recipes that would impress the heck out of you at a restaurant but is very little trouble to make for yourself at home.

    12 ounces (340 g) sea bass fillet

    3 tablespoons (45 ml) olive oil

    1/4 medium onion

    1/2 teaspoon minced garlic or 1 clove garlic, crushed

    2 tablespoons (16 g) tapenade

    1 tablespoon (15 ml) balsamic vinegar

    1 teaspoon lemon juice

    3 tablespoons (45 ml) heavy cream

    Salt and pepper

If the bass is in one piece, cut it into two equal portions. Brush with 1 tablespoon (15 ml) of the olive oil and put it under a broiler set on High, 3 or 4 inches (7.5 to 10 cm) from the heat. The length of time the fish will need to broil will depend on its thickness. I use fillets about 1 1/2-inch (3.8 cm) thick, and they take about 5 to 6 minutes per side.

While the fish is broiling, slice the quarter-onion in half lengthwise and then slice as thinly as possible. Put the rest of the olive oil in a medium-size skillet over medium heat and add the onion and garlic. Sauté together for 3 to 4 minutes. Add the tapenade, stir in, and sauté for a few more minutes. (Remember that somewhere in here you'll need to turn the fish!)

Now, stir the vinegar and lemon juice into the mixture in your skillet and let it cook down for 1 to 2 minutes. Stir in the cream and let the whole thing cook down for another minute.

When the fish is done, place it on two serving plates. Salt and pepper the sauce to taste, spoon over the fish, and then serve.

Yield: 2 servings, each with 4 grams of carbohydrates, a trace of fiber, and 32 grams of protein.

☉Jalapeño Lime Scallops

I served this as a first course at a little dinner party, and everyone agreed they'd never had a better scallop dish, even at a restaurant. A sterling example of how a few perfect ingredients can combine to make something greater than the sum of the parts. By the way, you can use sea scallops instead of bay scallops if you like, but since they're bigger, they'll take longer to cook.

4 tablespoons (55 g) butter

1 1/2 pounds (680 g) bay scallops

2 medium-size fresh jalapeños

3 tablespoons (45 ml) lime juice

3 tablespoons (3 g) chopped cilantro

Guar or xanthan

Melt the butter in a big, heavy skillet over medium heat. Add the scallops and sauté for a few minutes, stirring often. In the meanwhile, split the jalapeños lengthwise and remove the stems, seeds, and ribs. Slice them lengthwise again, into quarters, and then slice them as thin as you can crosswise. Add to the skillet and sauté the jalapenos with the scallops until the scallops are cooked through—they should look quite opaque all over. (And wash your hands! You must always wash your hands after handling hot peppers, or you'll be sorry the next time you touch your eyes, lips, or nose.)

Stir in the lime juice and cook for another minute while you chop the cilantro. Thicken the pan juices slightly with the guar or xanthan and divide the scallops between serving plates, spooning the pan juices over them. Scatter the cilantro on top and serve.

Yield: 4 main-dish servings or 6 first-course servings. Assuming 4 servings, each will have 6 grams of carbohydrates, a trace of fiber, and 29 grams of protein.

☉ Chili-Bacon Scallops

Bacon-wrapped scallops are a perennial favorite, but that whole wrapping thing blows past our time limit. Here's the easy solution: Just sauté the two together! Chili powder adds a little extra kick. You can use sea scallops if you prefer, but bay scallops, being smaller, cook faster.

> 8 slices bacon
>
> 1 pound (455 g) bay scallops
>
> 2 teaspoons chili powder

This is so simple! Put your big, heavy skillet over medium heat and snip the bacon into it in bits about 1/4 inch (6 mm) wide. Let that fry.

Sprinkle the chili powder all over the scallops; I sprinkled both sides and then stirred them up to make sure they were evenly seasoned.

When the bacon bits are about halfway to done, add the scallops to the skillet and spread them out in a single layer. Let them cook for about 5 minutes, turning them a few times, until they're done through and the bacon bits are crisp. Serve with the bacon bits and pour the grease over the top!

Yield: 3 to 4 servings, assuming 4, each will have 177 calories, 7 grams fat, 23 grams protein, 3 grams carbohydrate, trace dietary fiber, and 3 grams usable carb.

15~Minute Steaks and Chops

Steaks, chops, and other simple slabs of protein are classic fast low-carb fare, and let's face it, they're very nice simply broiled. But sometimes you want a little change. Here you'll find some quick-and-easy ways to add interest to these familiar foods.

⊕ Steak with Horseradish Butter

Horseradish is a classic accompaniment to beef.

> 1 steak, 12 to 16 ounces (340 to 455 g), well-marbled—sirloin, rib eye, strip steak, or the like
> 2 tablespoons (28 g) butter
> 1 to 2 teaspoons prepared horseradish
> Salt and pepper

Broil the steak as close to the flame as you can get it, with the broiler set on High. For a 1-inch thick (2.5 cm) steak, I like about 6 to 6 1/2 minutes per side, but you should experiment and cook it to your liking.

While the steak is broiling, put the butter and the horseradish in your food processor with the S-blade in place or in your blender, and run just long enough to blend. When the steak is done cooking, salt and pepper it, divide it into servings, and scoop a dollop of the horseradish butter on each serving.

Yield: 2 or 3 servings. Each 6-ounce (170 g) serving will have no more than 1 gram of carbohydrates, no fiber, and 24 grams of protein.

Note: Be careful when buying prepared horseradish! A lot of brands add sugar. Look for one that only contains grated horseradish root and vinegar. (I like Woeber's.)

☉ Orange Steak

This gives a nice tang to a simple grilled steak.

        3 tablespoons (45 ml) orange juice

        1 tablespoon (15 ml) dry sherry

        1 teaspoon soy sauce

        1 teaspoon Splenda

        1/2 teaspoon minced garlic or 1/2 clove garlic, crushed

        12 to 16 ounces (340 to 455 g) steak, 1/2 inch (1.3 cm) thick—rib eye, sirloin,
            strip steaks, or anything tender and fit for broiling

        Salt or Vege-Sal and pepper

Combine the orange juice, sherry, soy sauce, Splenda, and garlic. Put the steak on a plate, pour the orange juice mixture over it, and turn it over a few times to coat the whole surface. Let the steak sit for 2 to 3 minutes.

Now broil the steak as close as possible to a high flame until it's done to your liking—4 1/2 to 5 minutes per side is about right for me. Baste both sides with the orange mixture when you turn it! Salt, pepper, and serve.

Yield: The number of servings will depend on the size of your steak. Given a 12-ounce (355 g) steak, I'd call it 2 servings, each with 3 grams of carbohydrates, a trace of fiber, and 25 grams of protein.

☉ Costa Brava Steak

I was surprised that this traditional, anchovy-based Spanish sauce was not particularly fishy—just rich, mellow, and complex.

> 12 to 16 ounces (340 to 455 g) steak, 1/2- to 3/4-inch thick (1.3 to 1.9 cm)—rib eye, sirloin, strip, or anything tender and fit for broiling
>
> 1/3 cup (34 g) shelled walnuts
>
> 3 anchovy fillets
>
> 1/2 teaspoon red wine vinegar or sherry vinegar
>
> 1/3 cup (80 ml) olive oil

Start the steak broiling as close as possible to a high flame. Set your timer to remind you when to turn it—for a steak 1/2-inch thick (1.3 cm), 5 minutes per side is about right for my tastes.

While the steak is broiling, put the walnuts, anchovies, and vinegar in your food processor with the S-blade in place. Pulse to chop everything together—unless your machine is smaller than mine, the mixture will end up out against the walls of the processor bowl pretty quickly!

Scrape down the sides of the processor to get the mixture back into the path of the blade. Put the top back on, turn the processor on, and slowly pour in about half of the olive oil. If necessary, scrape down the sides of the processor again at this point and then turn it back on and add the rest of the oil.

When both sides of the steak are done, spread this sauce over the steak. Turn the broiler to Low, put the steak back under it for just a minute, and then serve.

Yield: The number of servings will depend on the size of your steak. Assuming a 12-ounce (340 g) steak, I'd call it 2 servings, each with 3 grams of carbohydrates and 1 gram of fiber, for a total of 2 grams of usable carbs and 31 grams of protein.

☉ Inauthentic Bulgogi Steak

True Bulgogi is a popular Korean dish made with very thin sheets of sliced beef. We don't have time in our 15 minutes to carefully slice up our beef, so we're using good old steak, and boy, are the results spectacular!

1/4 medium onion

2 teaspoons minced garlic or 4 cloves garlic, peeled

1/4 cup (60 ml) soy sauce

2 tablespoons (3 g) Splenda

1 teaspoon pepper

A few dashes Tabasco

2 tablespoons (28 ml) toasted sesame oil

1 1/2 pounds (680 g) tender, well-marbled steaks, 1/2-inch (1.3 cm) thick—sirloin, rib eye, strip, or whatever you like

Put the onion, garlic, soy sauce, Splenda, pepper, Tabasco, and sesame oil in a food processor with the S-blade in place and run it until the onion is pulverized.

Place the steaks on a plate and pour the seasoning mixture over them, turning them so that they're coated on both sides. Let the steaks sit for a minute and then place them on a broiler rack. Broil the steaks as close to a high flame as possible until they're done to your liking—4 1/2 to 5 minutes per side is right for me. When you're turning the steaks, spoon some of the seasoning mixture from the plate, first over the side that's already done and then over the side about to be broiled.

Yield: 4 servings. Calculations show 4 grams per serving and a trace of fiber, but that would only be true if you ate all of the seasoning mixture, which you won't. Figure closer to 2 grams of carbs and 26 grams of protein.

⊕ Steak Diane

This is actually a simplified version of a classic recipe—the original version didn't fit into our 15-minute time frame. It's really good, though!

12-ounce (340 g) steak, 1/2-inch (1.3 cm) thick*

2 tablespoons (28 g) butter

3 scallions, finely minced

1 tablespoon (4 g) minced fresh parsley

1 1/2 teaspoons minced garlic

1 tablespoon (15 ml) brandy

2 tablespoons (28 ml) dry sherry

1 1/2 teaspoons Worcestershire sauce

* Use rib eye, sirloin, strip, or whatever you like.

In a heavy skillet over medium-high heat, sauté the steak in the butter—figure 5 to 6 minutes per side. While that's happening, mince up the scallions and parsley.

When the steak is done to your liking, remove it to a platter and keep it warm. Turn the burner down to medium. Add the scallions, parsley, and garlic and sauté in the butter for a minute or so. Add the brandy, sherry, and Worcestershire sauce, turn the heat back up, and boil hard while stirring, to scrape any nice brown bits off the bottom of the pan. Let it boil for a minute or so to reduce, pour it over the steak, and serve.

Yield: 2 servings, each with 3 grams of carbohydrates and 2 grams of fiber, for a total of just 1 gram of usable carbs and 25 grams of protein.

☉ Many-Pepper Steak

This is so good! Make the *Cumin Mushrooms* (see page 265) as a side and toss some bagged salad with ranch or vinaigrette, and you're livin' large—without gettin' large!

> 12-ounce (340 g) steak, 1/2-inch (1.3 cm) thick*
>
> *Many-Pepper Steak Seasoning* (see page 302)

* I think rib eye is best for this, but it's not essential; use what you like.

Sprinkle both sides of the steak liberally with the *Many-Pepper Steak Seasoning*—about 1 teaspoon per side—and broil close to the flame until done to your liking (5 minutes per side is about right for me).

Yield: 2 servings, each with 3 grams of carbohydrates and 1 gram of fiber, for a total of 2 grams of usable carbs and 25 grams of protein.

⊕ Pan-Broiled Steak

This is a method rather than a recipe, but it's become our favorite way of cooking a steak. It's quicker than broiling and makes for a crustier outside. Don't worry about the measurements much, by the way; I just included them because they were needed for a nutritional breakdown. You know steak's got no carbs, so don't worry.

> 1 ½ pounds (680 g) steak, 1-inch (2.5 cm) thick—We like rib eye, but T-bone, sirloin, or strip will all do.
>
> 1 tablespoon bacon grease (15 g) or olive oil (15 ml)

Put your big, heavy skillet—cast iron is best—over highest heat and let it get good and hot. In the meantime, you can season your steak if you like. We like the *Montreal Steak Seasoning* that's currently popular, or you could use *Southwestern Steak Rub* on page 306 or the *Cocoa-Chili Rub* on page 307—anything you like. Or instead, you could top it when done with the *Bacon-Butter* on page 297, or butter and blue cheese, or sautéed onions and mushrooms, or go for classic simplicity and just salt and pepper it.

When the skillet's hot, add the bacon grease or oil and slosh it around and then throw in your steak. Set a timer for 5 to 6 minutes—your timing will depend on your taste and how hot your burner gets, but on my stove, 5 minutes per side with a 1-inch (2.5 cm) thick steak comes out medium rare. When the timer goes off, flip the steak and set the timer again. When time is up, devour immediately!

Yield: 4 servings, each with 403 calories, 33 grams fat, 24 grams protein, 0 grams carbohydrate, 0 grams dietary fiber, and 0 grams usable carb.

⊕Rib Eye Steak with Wine Sauce

This is a classic.

> 1 tablespoon (15 ml) olive oil
>
> 1 1/2 pounds (680 g) beef rib eye
>
> 2 shallots
>
> 1/2 cup (120 ml) dry red wine
>
> 1/2 cup (120 ml) beef stock, or 1/2 cup (120 ml) water and 1/2 teaspoon beef bouillon concentrate
>
> 1 tablespoon (15 ml) balsamic vinegar
>
> 1 teaspoon brown mustard, or Dijon
>
> 1 tablespoon (4 g) dried thyme
>
> 3 tablespoons (42 g) butter
>
> salt and pepper to taste

Cook your steak as described in *Pan Broiled Steak*.

In the meantime, assemble everything for your wine sauce—chop your shallots and measure the wine, beef stock, vinegar, mustard, and thyme together in a measuring cup with a pouring lip. Whisk them up.

When the timer goes off, flip the steak and set the timer again.

When your steak is done, put it on a platter. Pour the wine mixture into the skillet and stir it around, scraping up the nice brown bits, and let it boil hard. Continue boiling your sauce until it's reduced by at least half. Melt in the butter, salt and pepper, and serve with your steak.

Yield: 4 servings, each with 428 calories, 28 grams fat, 35 grams protein, 2 grams carbohydrate, trace dietary fiber, and 2 grams usable carb.

⊕ Beef and Blue Rollups

This makes a nice, cool supper for a hot night. If you cut the rolls in pieces, they'd make good party food, too. Warning: My ingredients didn't come out exactly even, and yours may not either.

1 jarred roasted red pepper, drained

1 bunch watercress

1/2 small red onion, minced

1/3 cup (75 g) mayonnaise

1 teaspoon prepared horseradish

1 pound (455 g) sliced deli roast beef, not too thin

6 ounces (90 g) crumbled blue cheese

Drain your roasted red pepper and cut it into strips. Chop your watercress and red onion together; you can do this in your food processor if you like, but I didn't bother. If you do, put the onion in and pulse a few times before you add the watercress or the watercress will be pulp before the onion is fine.

Mix the mayo and the horseradish together.

Okay, it's assembly line time: Lay a slice of roast beef on your cutting board. Spread it edge-to-edge with the horseradish mayo, sprinkle it evenly with some blue cheese, and then sprinkle with onion and watercress. Place a strip of roasted red pepper across one narrow edge and roll the whole thing up around it. Repeat the process until you run out of ingredients! I got about a dozen rolls. I don't guarantee your ingredients will come out exactly even because I don't know how thickly sliced your roast beef is, which will determine how many rolls you'll get.

Yield: I got 12 rolls, each with 164 calories, 11 grams fat, 14 grams protein, 3 grams carbohydrate, trace dietary fiber, and 3 grams usable carb.

About Lamb Steaks

Everybody's heard of lamb chops, but lamb steaks are harder to find. However, I think they're better and I can get them cheaper than most lamb chops, too. Here's how: I wait until whole legs of lamb are on sale at my grocery store—at least a few times a year they go as low as $3.99 a pound. When they do, I buy one or two, and have the meat guy at the grocery store slice a smallish roast off either end (these make far more sense for small households than a whole leg of lamb), and slice the center into steaks 1/2 inch (1.3 cm) thick. I've never been charged for this service. When I get them home, I bag everything up and stash it in the freezer—where they don't last very long, since I'm hopelessly devoted to lamb!

However, if you prefer, you can make any of these lamb recipes with 1/2-inch thick (1.3 cm) lamb chops, instead.

☉ Soy and Sesame Glazed Lamb Steaks

 2 lamb steaks, 6 to 8 ounces (170 to 225 g) each, 1/2-inch (1.3 cm) thick

 2 tablespoons (28 ml) olive oil

 1 teaspoon minced garlic or 2 cloves garlic, crushed

 2 scallions, minced

 2 tablespoons (28 ml) soy sauce

 1 teaspoon Splenda

 6 drops or 1/4 teaspoon blackstrap molasses*

 2 teaspoons sesame oil

* I keep my molasses in a squeeze container to make it easy to measure out very small quantities.

In a heavy skillet, start sautéing the lamb steaks in the oil over high heat. Cook for 5 to 6 minutes per side.

While the lamb is browning, prepare and combine the garlic, scallions, soy sauce, Splenda, molasses, and sesame oil.

Remove the lamb from the skillet, add the soy sauce mixture, and stir a bit. Replace the lamb in the skillet, turn it once to coat with sauce, and cook it for another 1 to 2 minutes per side. Serve, scraping the liquid from the pan over the lamb steaks.

Yield: 2 servings. Assuming each steak is 6 ounces (170 g), each will have 4 grams of carbohydrates and 1 gram of fiber, for a total of 3 grams of usable carbs and 23 grams of protein.

⊕ Curried Lamb Steak

    2 tablespoons (28 g) butter

    2 teaspoons curry powder

    1 teaspoon minced garlic or 2 cloves garlic, crushed

    2 lamb steaks, 6 to 8 ounces (170 to 225 g) each, 1/2 inch (1.3 cm) thick

Melt the butter in large, heavy skillet over medium heat. Add the curry powder and garlic, stir, and add the lamb steak. Cover with a tilted lid and cook for 7 minutes. Turn, recover with a tilted lid, and cook for another 7 minutes. Remove the lamb to serving plates, scrape the curry butter over the steaks, and serve.

Yield: 2 servings. Assuming each steak is 6 ounces, each will have 2 grams of carbohydrates and 1 gram of fiber, for a total of 1 gram of usable carbs and 23 grams of protein.

⊕ Barbecued Lamb Steaks

    2 lamb steaks, 6 to 8 ounces each (170 to 225 g), 1/2-inch (1.3 cm) thick

    1 tablespoon (15 g) plus 1 teaspoon (5 g) sugar-free ketchup

    1 tablespoon (15 ml) plus 1 teaspoon (5 ml) cider vinegar

    1 tablespoon (15 ml) plus 1 teaspoon (5 ml) Worcestershire sauce

    1 teaspoon spicy brown mustard

Broil the lamb steaks close to the flame for 6 to 7 minutes. While the steaks are cooking, combine the ketchup, vinegar, Worcestershire sauce, and mustard.

Turn the steaks and broil the second side for 3 to 4 minutes. Spoon the sauce over the steaks and broil for another 2 to 3 minutes. Serve.

Yield: 2 servings. Assuming each steak is 6 ounces (170 g), each will have 4 grams of carbohydrates, a trace of fiber, and 23 grams of protein.

About Pork Loin

Whole pork loin is another largish cut of meat that often goes on sale at attractive prices. Again, if you buy a whole pork loin, the nice people behind the meat counter will be glad to cut it to your specifications. Keep in mind, however, that pork ages poorly in the freezer—use it up within two to three months, or it will taste nasty.

⊕ Pineapple Glazed Pork Loin

You can double this recipe if you like, but if your skillet's the size of mine, you'll have to cook it in two batches—which, of course, takes twice the time.

> 3/4 pound (340 g) boneless pork loin, cut about ¹/₂-inch (1.3 cm) thick*
>
> 1 to 2 tablespoons (15 to 28 ml) olive oil
>
> 2 tablespoons (30 g) canned, crushed pineapple in juice
>
> 2 teaspoons cider vinegar
>
> 2 teaspoons Splenda
>
> 1 teaspoon spicy brown or Dijon mustard
>
> ¹/₂ teaspoon soy sauce
>
> 1 teaspoon minced garlic or 2 cloves garlic, crushed

* Feel free to use thinish pork chops, instead.

First, pound the pork until it's about 1/4 inch (6 mm) thick. Heat the oil in a heavy skillet over medium-high heat and sauté the pork, covering it with a tilted lid. Give it 4 to 5 minutes per side.

While the pork's browning, combine the pineapple, vinegar, Splenda, mustard, soy sauce, and garlic. When the pork is browned on both sides, add this mixture to the skillet. Turn the pork over once or twice to coat. Put the tilted lid back on the pan, cook for 1 to 2 minutes, turn, re-cover, and give it another 1 to 2 minutes. Remove to serving plates and scrape any remaining liquid from the pan over the pork before serving.

Yield: 2 servings, each with 4 grams of carbohydrates, a trace of fiber, and 22 grams of protein.

☉ Chili Lime Pork Strips

I didn't know where else in the book to put this, but it was too good and too versatile to leave out! Use the strips for a Chili Lime Pork Salad or a Chili Lime Pork Omelet or just wrap them up in low-carb tortillas with a little salsa and sour cream.

1 pound (455 g) boneless pork loin

1 to 2 tablespoons (15 to 28 ml) oil

1 1/2 teaspoons chili powder

1 tablespoon (15 ml) lime juice

Slice the pork as thinly as you can into small strips (this is easier if the pork is half-frozen). Heat the oil in a large, heavy skillet over medium-high heat and add the pork. Stir-fry the pork strips until they're nearly done—about 6 to 7 minutes—then stir in the chili powder and lime juice. Continue stirring and cooking for another 3 to 4 minutes. These strips keep well for a few days in a closed container in the fridge.

Yield: 4 servings, each with 1 gram of carbohydrates, a trace of fiber, and 23 grams of protein.

⊕ Cherry Chops

An unusual sauce of tart cherries and a crunch of toasted almonds enhance these pork chops. Don't expect this sauce to be cherry-red, though, unless you add a drop or two of food coloring.

    4 thin pork chops, about 18 ounces (510 g) total
    Salt and pepper
    1 tablespoon (15 ml) olive oil
    1/2 cup (123 g) canned tart cherries in water (pie cherries)
    1 tablespoon (15 ml) wine vinegar
    1/4 teaspoon dry mustard
    1/8 teaspoon ground cloves
    1 1/2 tablespoons (2.3 g) Splenda
    1/8 teaspoon guar or xanthan
    1/3 cup (37 g) slivered almonds
    1/2 tablespoon butter

Salt and pepper the chops lightly on both sides and start browning them in the oil in a heavy skillet over medium-high heat. Give them about 5 minutes per side. While that's happening, put the cherries, vinegar, mustard, cloves, Splenda, and guar or xanthan in a blender and purée the whole thing together. (If you'd prefer to keep the cherries whole, you could just mix everything together well. I like it puréed.)

It's time to turn the chops now! While the chops are browning on their second side, start browning the almonds in the butter in a small skillet over medium heat. Stir frequently so they don't burn; you just want a touch of gold. When the almonds are toasted, don't forget to turn off the heat, and if you have an electric stove, remove the pan from the burner.

When the second side of the chops is browned—again, about 5 minutes—pour the cherry sauce over them, turn the burner to medium-low, and cover the skillet with a tilted lid. Let the whole thing simmer for 5 minutes and serve. Scrape the sauce from the skillet over the chops and top each with toasted almonds.

Yield: 4 servings, each with 6 grams of carbohydrates and 1 gram of fiber, for a total of 5 grams of usable carbs and 22 grams of protein.

☺ Gingersnap Pork

Okay, it doesn't really have gingersnaps in it, but it is sweet and spicy and good!

4 thin pork chops, about 18 ounces (510 g) total

1 tablespoon (15 ml) olive oil

1/2 cup (120 ml) cider vinegar

1/2 teaspoon pepper

1/4 teaspoon ground cloves

1 tablespoon (16 g) tomato paste

3 tablespoons (4.5 g) Splenda

2 teaspoons grated gingerroot

2 teaspoons lemon juice

1/2 teaspoon salt or Vege-Sal

1/4 cup (25 g) finely diced celery, including leaves

In a heavy skillet over medium-high heat, start browning the chops in the oil. While that's happening, put the vinegar, pepper, cloves, tomato paste, Splenda, gingerroot, lemon juice, and Vege-Sal in a blender and run it for a second or two to blend.

When the chops are browned on both sides—about 5 minutes per side—pour the sauce over them, scatter the celery over the whole thing, turn the burner to low, and cover with a tilted lid. Let it simmer for 5 minutes and then serve. Don't forget to scrape the extra sauce out of the pan and over the chops!

Yield: 4 servings, each with 5 grams of carbohydrates, a trace of fiber, and 20 grams of protein.

◷ Pork Chops with Fennel and Gin

Fennel looks a bit like celery, but with feathery leaves and a swollen bulb at the base. Some markets label it "anise." For this recipe we use the bulb, but if you like you can save the leaves for salad, or to use as garnish.

> 12 ounces (340 g) pork chops, no more than 1/2 inch (1.3 cm) thick
>
> salt and pepper
>
> 2 tablespoons (28 ml) olive oil
>
> 1/2 fennel bulb
>
> 1 tablespoon (15 ml) rice vinegar
>
> 1 tablespoon (15 ml) lemon juice
>
> 3 drops orange extract
>
> 1 teaspoon Splenda, or liquid Splenda to equal a teaspoon of sugar
>
> 1 tablespoon (15 ml) gin

Put your big, heavy skillet over high heat. While it's heating, sprinkle your chops both sides with salt and pepper.

When the skillet's hot, add the oil and slosh it around to coat the bottom of the skillet. Add the chops; keep the heat high. You want them to brown a little on both sides.

In the meantime, sliced your fennel lengthwise as thinly as possible. Flip your chops! Now, in a small dish, mix the vinegar, lemon juice, orange extract, Splenda, and gin.

When your chops are browned a bit on both sides, remove them from the skillet, add the fennel in an even layer over the bottom, and lay the chops on top. Cover with a tilted lid for five minutes or so.

Add the vinegar-lemon juice-gin mixture and re-cover with the tilted lid for the remaining time. Serve the chops with the fennel and pan liquid on top.

Yield: 2 servings each with 423 calories, 30 grams fat, 27 grams protein, 6 grams carbohydrate, 2 grams dietary fiber, and 4 grams usable carb.

About Pork Steaks

Shoulder steaks are my favorite cut of pork—I think they're juicier and more flavorful than pork loin or most chops, probably because they have more fat! Pork steaks have a lot of advantages for the low-carber in a hurry—they cook quickly, they're often quite cheap, and they take to a variety of easy seasonings, so you can vary them at will. Here are the two ways I most often cook pork steaks, plus a very slightly more complicated bonus recipe.

⊕ Sautéed Pork Steak

Pork steaks vary considerably in size. Whether you have a single-serving pork steak or a two-serving pork steak will depend on the size of your steak, not to mention the size of your appetite. Feel free to do two steaks at a time if they'll fit in your skillet.

> Olive oil
>
> Pork shoulder steak, no more than 1/2-inch (1.3 cm) thick
>
> Sprinkle-on seasoning of your choice—Cajun, Creole, Soul, Barbecue,
>   and Jerk seasonings are all great used this way.

Heat a heavy skillet over medium-high heat. Add the olive oil, slosh it around, and throw in the pork steak. Sprinkle the top with the sprinkle-on seasoning. Let the steak cook for about 7 minutes or until it's well-browned and a bit crusty on the bottom. Flip it, sprinkle the seasoning on the cooked side, and let it cook for another 7 minutes or until well-browned on the second side and cooked through. Serve.

Yield: How many servings this makes will depend—as noted—on how big your steak is. I can eat a medium-size pork steak all by myself, and I often do! The sprinkle-on seasoning is unlikely to add more than 1 gram of carbs per serving, but do read your labels and choose brands with little or no sugar or make your own.

Note: Instead of sprinkle-on seasoning, you can add some minced garlic toward the end and flip the steak once or twice to flavor both sides. Don't add the garlic right at the beginning, though; it's liable to burn and go bitter on you.

⊕ Grilled Pork Steak

Cooking your pork steaks in your electric tabletop grill cuts the cooking time down to 7 to 8 minutes. The trade-off is that your steak will be less browned and crusty than if you'd done it in a skillet.

> Pork shoulder steak, no more than 1/2 inch (1.3 cm) thick
>
> Sprinkle-on seasoning—Cajun, Creole, Soul, Barbecue, and Jerk seasonings
>   are all good used this way.

Preheat your electric tabletop grill.

While it's heating, lay the steak on a plate and sprinkle both sides liberally with the seasoning of your choice. When the grill is hot, throw the pork steak in and give it 7 to 8 minutes or until it's cooked through. Serve.

Yield: Again, how many servings this makes depends on the size of your steak, but the carb count is unlikely to be more than 1 gram, even if you eat the whole thing.

⊕Mustard-Maple Glazed Pork Steak

I rarely tire of pork steaks with just a little Cajun seasoning or barbecue rub, but this is very little more trouble and seriously tasty.

> 2 pounds (900 g) pork shoulder, steaks, no more than 1/2-inch (1.3 cm) thick
>
> salt and pepper
>
> 1 tablespoon (15 ml) olive oil
>
> 1/4 cup (60 ml) chicken broth or 1/4 cup (60 ml) water and 1/4 teaspoon chicken bouillon granules
>
> 1 tablespoon (20 g) sugar-free pancake syrup
>
> 1 tablespoon (11 g) spicy brown or Dijon mustard

Give your big, heavy skillet a shot of nonstick cooking spray and start it heating over high heat while you salt and pepper the pork steaks. In a minute or so, add the olive oil, slosh it around to coat the pan, and throw in your steaks. Cover them with a tilted lid.

Mix together everything else and place by the stove.

After about five minutes, flip your pork steaks and let them cook on the other side, again with a tilted lid.

With about 3 minutes left, transfer the steaks to a plate. Pour the mustard-maple mixture into the pan and stir it around, scraping up any tasty brown bits. Let it boil hard until it cooks down by about half. Put the steaks back in and flip them to coat and let the whole thing keep cooking just a minute more until the sauces is about the texture of half-and-half. Plate the steaks, pour the sauce over them, and serve.

Yield: 4 servings, each with 437 calories, 34 grams fat, 30 grams protein, 1 grams carbohydrate, trace dietary fiber, and 1 gram usable carb.

⊕ Maple-Chipotle Glaze Glazed Pork Steaks

 2 pounds (900 g) pork shoulder steaks or pork chops, no more than 1/2-inch
   (1.3 cm) thick

 1 tablespoon bacon grease (15 g) or coconut oil (15 ml)

 1/3 cup (107 g) sugar-free pancake syrup

 2 to 3 chipotle chiles canned in adobo

 1 1/2 teaspoons adobo sauce

 1 1/2 teaspoons spicy brown mustard

 1 teaspoon chopped garlic

Put your big, heavy skillet over medium-high heat and start the pork steaks browning in the bacon grease or oil.

Throw everything else in your blender or food processor and run until the chipotles and garlic are pulverized. Store in a tightly lidded container in the fridge.

When your steaks are browned on both sides, add the glaze to the skillet and flip the steaks to coat on both sides. Cover with a tilted lid and let it cook until the steaks are done through and the glaze has cooked down a little. Serve with all the glaze scraped over the steaks.

Yield: 4 servings, each with 434 calories, 32 grams fat, 32 grams protein, 3 grams carbohydrate, 1 gram dietary fiber, and 2 grams usable carb.

⊕ Pork Crusted Pork!

> 8 ounces (225 g) pork shoulder steak, 1/2-inch (1.3 cm) thick
>
> 1/3 cup (80 g) crushed barbecue-flavor pork rinds
>
> 1 to 2 tablespoons (15 to 28 ml) oil

Coat both sides of the pork steak with the crushed pork rinds. (It's easiest to spread the crushed pork rinds on a plate and press each side of the pork steak into them.) Heat the oil in a heavy skillet over medium-high heat and sauté the steak until it's crisp on both sides and cooked through—about 7 minutes per side.

Yield: 1 or 2 servings. There are no carbohydrates or fiber here at all, and the whole steak will have about 45 grams of protein.

Bacon

⊕ Maple-Glazed Bacon

I know, I know, this is really a side dish. But it didn't really belong with the veggies and noodles and such, and it is pork, after all. It makes a great, festive treat for a holiday breakfast.

> 6 bacon slices
>
> 1/4 cup (80 g) sugar-free pancake syrup

Simply brush the bacon with the pancake syrup on both sides before laying it on a microwave bacon rack or in a Pyrex pie plate. Nuke on high for 8 minutes and then check—it may well need a few more minutes; I discovered that for some reason bacon cooks more slowly with the syrup on it. It may take 10 to 11 minutes to crisp, depending on your microwave.

Yield: Each slice will have 41 calories, 3 grams fat, 2 grams protein, 1 grams carbohydrate, 0 grams dietary fiber, and 1 gram usable carb.

15~Minute Main Dish Salads

Main dish salads are one of the greatest ways to eat low carb. They're quick, simple, delicious, beautiful to look at, offer endless variety, and pack more nutrition into a single meal than most anything else you can think of. I hope you'll serve these main dish salads often, especially on hot summer days—and nights.

Here are some new ideas to take you beyond your old standby tuna salad and the ubiquitous chicken Caesar.

⊕ Tomatoes with Pecans, Basil, and Cheese

Originally I thought of this as a first course, but it's darned filling and has as much protein per serving as a couple of eggs, so I put it here. Still, it would make a nice starter if your main course is light.

> 1/2 cup (50 g) pecan halves
>
> 2 tablespoons (28 ml) olive oil
>
> 1/3 cup (80 ml) olive oil
>
> 1/3 cup (80 ml) red wine vinegar
>
> 1/4 cup (6 g) Splenda, or equivalent in liquid sucralose
>
> 1 clove garlic, crushed
>
> 1/4 teaspoon pepper
>
> 1/2 teaspoon salt

1 cup (40 g) fresh basil leaves

2 scallions

1 cup (115 g) 6 cheese Italian blend, the finely shredded kind

2 big ripe tomatoes

In a heavy skillet over low-medium heat, start the pecan halves toasting in the 2 tablespoons (28 ml) of olive oil.

In the meantime, measure the 1/3 (80 ml) cup olive oil, vinegar, Splenda, garlic, pepper, and salt and whisk together. Don't forget to take a break to stir your pecans so they don't scorch!

Okay, pecans are toasted and dressing is made. Transfer your pecans to your food processor with the S-blade in place. Add the basil. Trim the root and any limp part of the green shoot off the scallions, whack each into three or four pieces, and throw them in, too. Now pulse until everything's chopped medium-fine.

Dump your pecan mixture into a small mixing bowl, add the shredded cheese, and toss everything together.

Slice your tomatoes and divide the slices between four plates, arranging them prettily. Sprinkle the pecan-cheese mixture evenly over them, drizzle with the dressing, and serve.

Yield: 4 servings, each with 525 calories, 49 grams fat, 17 grams protein, 11 grams carbohydrate, 2 grams dietary fiber, and 9 grams usable carb.

☉Tuna Salad with Lemon and Capers

I've always loved the bright, sunny flavors of lemon and capers in foods cooked "piccata." This is my way of adding those Mediterranean flavors to tuna salad.

> 1 can (5 ounces, or 140 g) tuna, drained
> 1/2 cup (80 g) diced sweet red onion (50 g)
> 2 stalks celery, diced
> 1/3 cup (20 g) chopped parsley
> 1 tablespoon (9 g) capers
> 1 tablespoon (15 ml) lemon juice
> 1 tablespoon (15 ml) olive oil
> 1 tablespoon (14 ml) mayonnaise

Just drain the tuna, put it in a bowl with the onion, celery, parsley, and capers, and mix. Add the lemon juice, olive oil, and mayonnaise and stir it together until it's thoroughly combined. It's nice to serve this on a bed of lettuce, but it's not essential.

Yield: 2 servings, each with 5 grams of carbohydrates and 2 grams of fiber, for a total of 3 grams of usable carbs and 19 grams of protein.

✫ It's only 214 calories per serving if you use water packed tuna.

☉ Curried Tuna Salad

This is good as-is or as an omelet filling (see page 37).

> 1/2 cup (55 g) slivered almonds
>
> 2 tablespoons (28 g) plus 1/2 teaspoon butter
>
> 1 large stalk celery, diced
>
> 1 scallion, sliced
>
> I can (6 ounces, or 170 g) tuna, drained
>
> 2 tablespoons (30 g) sour cream
>
> 2 tablespoons (28 g) mayonnaise
>
> 1 tablespoon (15 ml) lemon juice
>
> 1/8 teaspoon pepper
>
> 3/4 teaspoon curry powder

Sauté the almonds in 2 tablespoons (28 g) of butter over medium-high heat, stirring frequently, until the almonds are golden. Remove from the heat and set aside.

Dice the celery and slice the scallion, open and drain the tuna, and combine them all in a mixing bowl. Add the sour cream, mayo, lemon juice, and pepper.

In your smallest skillet, melt the last 1/2 teaspoon of butter and sauté the curry powder in it, over medium heat, for just a minute (this brings out the full flavor of the curry). Scrape the curry butter into the salad and mix until the curry is well-distributed throughout. Stir in the almonds and serve.

Yield: If you serve this as a salad—over a bed of greens is nice—this makes 2 servings, each with 6 grams of carbohydrates and 2 grams of fiber, for a total of 4 grams of usable carbs and 22 grams of protein.

⊕ Tuna "Rice" Salad

Can you tell I like tuna?

> 1/2 head cauliflower
>
> 1 can (5 ounces, or 140 g) tuna
>
> 2 tablespoons (28 ml) lime juice
>
> 1 can (2 1/2 ounces, or 70 g) sliced ripe olives, drained
>
> 1 can (14 ounces, or 390 g) quartered artichoke hearts, drained
>
> 1/2 cup (115 g) mayonnaise
>
> 1 teaspoon dried dill weed

Run the cauliflower through the shredding blade of your food processor. Put it in a microwaveable casserole with a lid, add a couple of tablespoons (28 to 45 ml) of water, cover, and nuke on High for 7 minutes.

While that's happening, combine the tuna, lime juice, olives, artichoke hearts, mayonnaise, and dill. When the cauliflower is done, pull it out of the microwave, drain it, and toss it in with everything else.

Obviously, if you don't like a warm salad, you'll have to chill this—but that takes more than 15 minutes! And it sure tastes good warm. If you really want it cooled quickly, you could put the cauliflower "rice" in a strainer and run cold water over it for a minute.

Yield: 3 servings, each with 12 grams of carbohydrates and 1 gram of fiber, for a total of 11 grams of usable carbs and 16 grams of protein.

⊕ San Diego Tuna Salad

Yes, you really can get all of this—including the *Guacamole Dressing*—done in 15 minutes!

1 batch Guacamole Dressing (see page 298)

12 cups (684 g) bagged mixed greens

2/3 cup (70 g) sliced ripe olives

1/2 cup (80 g) diced sweet red onion

1 cup (70 g) sliced mushrooms

8 tablespoons (8 g) chopped cilantro

8 tablespoons (17 g) alfalfa sprouts

3 cans (5 ounces, or 140 g) tuna, drained

2 small tomatoes, cut into thin wedges

Make the *Guacamole Dressing* first.

In a large salad bowl, combine the mixed greens, olives, onion, mushrooms, cilantro and sprouts. Pour on the *Guacamole Dressing* and toss thoroughly.

Pile the salad on 4 or 5 serving plates. Top each serving with drained tuna and decorate each serving with tomato wedges. Serve.

Yield: 4 or 5 servings. Assuming 5 servings, each will have 14 grams of carbohydrates and 6 grams of fiber, for a total of 8 grams of usable carbs and 27 grams of protein.

✳ This salad also contains 1059 milligrams of potassium and less than 350 calories if you use water packed tuna.

⏲ Old Days Tuna Noodle Salad

Back when I believed whole grains were better for me than animal protein and fat, I used to make huge vats of salad using whole wheat elbow noodles, with lots of celery, onion, and apple, but just one can of tuna, plus a chopped egg and mayonnaise—low fat, of course! I could live on this for days. I thought it would be fun to come up with a version using shirataki.

1 packet tofu shirataki, fettucini style

2 celery ribs

3 scallions

1 apple

2 hard-boiled eggs

1 can (7 ounces, or 200 g) tuna

1/4 cup (60 g) mayonnaise

2 tablespoons (10 g) grated Parmesan cheese

Snip open your packet of shirataki and dump them into a strainer. Rinse, drain well, snip across them a few times with your kitchen shears, and throw them in a big mixing bowl.

Dice your celery and apple and slice the scallions (include the crisp part of the green shoot). Add to the mixing bowl. Peel and chop your eggs and throw them in there too.

Drain your tuna and add it to the mix. Measure in the mayo and Parmesan and mix the whole thing up. That's it! Serve on lettuce, if you like, but it's not essential.

Yield: 2 servings, each with 467 calories, 31 grams fat, 35 grams protein, 14 grams carbohydrate, 3 grams dietary fiber, and 11 grams usable carb.

Note: I use the chunk light tuna rather than the solid white. Not only is it cheaper, but it's far less likely to be contaminated with mercury.

☺ Debbie's Tuna-Cottage Cheese Scoops

My friend Debbie told me that she loved tuna mixed with cottage cheese, and "lots and lots of chopped dill pickles." So I tried it, and it made a really nice, simple lunch. This would travel well in a snap-top container, along with a baggie full of vegetables for scooping.

> 1 can (5 ounces, or 140 g) tuna, drained
>
> 1/2 cup (115 g) small-curd cottage cheese
>
> 1/4 cup (60 g) chopped dill pickle
>
> 1/4 cup (40 g) diced sweet red onion
>
> 1 tablespoon (14 g) mayonnaise
>
> Celery sticks, pepper strips, and/or cucumber rounds

Simply mix together the tuna, cottage cheese, dill pickle, red onion, and mayonnaise. Refrigerate until you're ready to eat it and then scoop the tuna-cottage cheese salad up with the veggies!

Yield: 2 servings. Exclusive of the vegetables used for scooping, each serving will have 5 grams of carbohydrates and 1 gram of fiber, for a total of 4 grams of usable carbs and 26 grams of protein.

⊕ Crabamole Salad

Even if you're making the *Guacamole Dressing* right then, this is incredibly quick and easy. Feel free to substitute the seafood of your choice for the crab—flaked, cooked lobster or small salad shrimp would work well. Just don't use fake seafood, such as "Delicaseas"—the stuff has a whole pile of added carbs.

> 24 ounces (680 g) bagged mixed greens
> 1 pound (455 g) cooked lump crabmeat
> 1 batch *Guacamole Dressing* (see page 298)
> 16 cherry tomatoes

Arrange the mixed greens on 4 serving plates. Top each with crabmeat and then top that with the *Guacamole Dressing*, letting it run artistically down onto the greens. Cut the cherry tomatoes in half and arrange them around each portion. Serve.

Yield: 4 servings, each with 17 grams of carbohydrates and 8 grams of fiber, for a total of 9 grams of usable carbs and 28 grams of protein.

⭐ There's also 1479 milligrams of potassium and 344 milligrams of calcium in each serving of this salad!

☉Thai-Style Crab Salad in Avocados

Short on time, I got my pal Julie McIntosh to try out this recipe for me. She loved it the way I'd conceived of it, but suggested a little more cilantro, plus a little scallion, so that's what we did. Thanks, Julie!

1 ripe avocado

3 tablespoons (45 ml) lime juice

1 can (6 ounces, or 170 g) crabmeat, or 6 ounces (170 g) cooked lump crabmeat

1 teaspoon lemon juice

1/4 cup (60 g) mayonnaise

2 tablespoons (2 g) chopped cilantro

1 scallion, thinly sliced

1/4 teaspoon pepper, or to taste

Salt, if desired

Split the avocado in half, remove the seed, and sprinkle the cut surfaces with 1 tablespoon (15 ml) of the lime juice to prevent browning.

Combine the crabmeat, remaining lemon juice, mayonnaise, cilantro, scallion, pepper, and salt in a mixing bowl and mix well. Stuff into the avocado halves, piling it high. Garnish with extra cilantro, if desired, and serve.

Yield: 2 servings, each with 9 grams of carbohydrates and 5 grams of fiber, for a total of 4 grams of usable carbs and 20 grams of protein.

✳ This salad also provides 932 milligrams of potassium and 110 milligrams of calcium.

⊕ Smoked Salmon and Blue Cheese Salad

This salad is super easy but elegant enough for an alfresco summer company lunch. It's also very simple to double or even triple.

> 1 pound (455 g) bagged romaine mix
>
> 1/3 cup (80 ml) bottled Dijon vinaigrette dressing
>
> 8 ounces (225 g) smoked salmon, flaked
>
> 3/4 cup (90 g) crumbled blue cheese
>
> 6 scallions, sliced
>
> 1/4 cup (25 g) chopped Smokehouse almonds

Put the romaine mix in a big salad bowl and toss well with the dressing. Pile the greens on 3 plates, top with the salmon, blue cheese, scallions, and almonds, in that order, and then serve.

Yield: 3 servings, each with 10 grams of carbohydrates and 5 grams of fiber, for a total of 5 grams of usable carbs and 26 grams of protein.

⊕ Shrimp and Spinach Caesar Salad

Traditionally, Caesar Salad is made with romaine, but raw spinach is delicious, fabulous for you, and makes a pretty contrast with the shrimp and the eggs. If you don't have hard-boiled eggs on hand in the refrigerator, feel free to leave them out. (But why don't you have hard-boiled eggs on hand in the refrigerator?)

> 1 pound (455 g) bagged, triple-washed baby spinach leaves
>
> 1/3 cup (80 ml) bottled Caesar dressing
>
> 8 ounces (225 g) cooked, peeled, bitsy little shrimp, either canned (drain first) or frozen (thaw them!)
>
> 2 hard-boiled eggs
>
> 3 tablespoons (15 g) shredded Parmesan cheese

Place the spinach in a big salad bowl, pour the dressing over it, and toss with reckless abandon until every square millimeter of every leaf is coated. Pile the spinach on 3 serving plates.

Divide the shrimp between the 3 plates, piling them in the middles of the beds of spinach.

Peel and slice the eggs and arrange the slices around each pile of shrimp. Scatter 1 tablespoon (15 g) of Parmesan over each salad and serve.

Yield: 3 servings, each with 7 grams of carbohydrates and 3 grams of fiber, for a total of 4 grams of usable carbs and 27 grams of protein.

⭐ You'll also get 238 milligrams of calcium and a whopping 821 milligrams of potassium!

☻ Not-Quite-Middle-Eastern Salad Plus

Add protein to this fabulous side dish salad and it becomes a very posh summer lunch or supper.

> 1 batch *Not-Quite-Middle-Eastern Salad* (see page 242)
> 1 pound (455 g) cooked crabmeat, lobster, or tiny shrimp

Make the salad according to the instructions and then toss in the shellfish. Serve on a bed of lettuce.

Yield: 4 servings, each with 7 grams of carbohydrates and 3 grams of fiber, for a total of 4 grams of usable carbs and 22 grams of protein.

☉ Egg Salad Francais

This is completely different from any egg salad you've ever had and quite wonderful! This is actually a French tradition.

8 ounces (225 g) bagged European style salad*

2 scallions, sliced

1/3 cup (80 ml) bottled balsamic vinaigrette—I like Paul Newman's.

Salt and pepper

1/4 cup (20 g) shredded Parmesan cheese**

1 tablespoon (15 ml) vinegar

4 very fresh eggs

* The mixture should include some frizee, so read the label! If you can't find one with frizee, you can still make the salad, but it will be less authentic.

** It is very important to use good-quality shredded (not grated) Parmesan with no additives. Regular Parmesan in the round green shaker won't work; the cellulose in it messes it up for this.

First put 1 inch (2.5 cm) of water in a largish saucepan and put it over a burner set to medium-high. Ignore that for a minute while you put the greens and scallions in a big salad bowl. Pour the vinaigrette over the whole thing, add salt and pepper as desired, and toss well. Set aside.

Spray a microwaveable plate with nonstick cooking spray and spread the Parmesan on it. Microwave on High for 1 minute.

While the cheese is nuking, let's get back to that water. It should be good and hot by now; turn it down to barely a simmer, add a tablespoon (15 ml) of vinegar, and poach the eggs in it. It helps to break each egg into a small cup or dish first to make sure that it's good and fresh and that the yolk doesn't break. (If it does, keep it for something else and use another egg for poaching.) Then slide each egg gently into the water and poach to the desired degree of doneness.

While the eggs are poaching, remove the Parmesan from the microwave—it will now be a crispy, lacy sheet. Break it up. Pile the salad on 2 serving plates and top each one with crispy Parmesan bits. Lift the now-poached eggs out of the pan with a slotted spoon, place 2 on each salad, and serve.

Yield: 2 servings, each with 10 grams of carbohydrates and 4 grams of fiber, for a total of 6 grams of usable carbs and 20 grams of protein.

⊙ Artichoke-Egg Lettuce Wraps

I just love lettuce wraps! Add some eggs and artichokes, and I'm a very happy girl.

1 jar (12 ounces, or 340 g) marinated artichoke hearts

1/4 cup (40 g) diced red onion

1/4 cup (15 g) chopped fresh parsley

2 tablespoons (28 ml) extra virgin olive oil

1 1/2 teaspoons lemon juice

salt and pepper

4 hard-boiled eggs

10 lettuce leaves—I like butter lettuce with this, but romaine would be fine

Drain the artichoke hearts and chop coarsely. Throw them in a mixing bowl. Dice up the onion, chop the parsley, and throw them in, too. Stir in the olive oil and lemon juice, plus salt and pepper to taste.

Peel your hard boiled eggs. Now mound half of the artichoke mixture on each of two plates and arrange 4 to 5 nice big lettuce leaves and two sliced hard boiled eggs next to it.

To eat, spoon artichoke mixture into a lettuce leaf, top with egg, wrap, and eat.

Yield: 2 servings, each with 442 calories, 33 grams fat, 20 grams protein, 17 grams carbohydrate, 7 grams dietary fiber, and 10 grams usable carb.

⊕ Egg and Avocado Salad

The key to this is to use an avocado that's just a little underripe and to mix gently.

> 3 hard-boiled eggs
>
> 3 tablespoons (30 g) minced red onion
>
> 10 sugar-free bread and butter pickle chips
>
> 2 tablespoons (28 g) mayonnaise
>
> 1 tablespoon (11 g) brown mustard
>
> 1 avocado, the little black kind
>
> salt and pepper to taste

Peel and chop the eggs and throw them in a mixing bowl. Mince your red onion, chop your pickles, and throw them in, too.

Add the mayo and mustard and stir the whole thing up.

Now peel and dice your avocado and stir it in gently; you're trying to keep it in cubes. Salt and pepper to taste.

You can serve this a number of ways: wrap it in lettuce leaves, use a low carb tortilla or Lavash, or stuff it into a tomato. Or you can do what I did: Eat it with a fork. It's yummy.

Yield: 2 servings, each with 396 calories, 36 grams fat, 13 grams protein, 11 grams carbohydrate, 3 grams dietary fiber, and 8 grams usable carb.

Note: Sugar-free bread and butter pickles are pretty easy to find; my local Kroger carries two brands: Mt. Olive and a house brand. Either is fine. Since Kroger is the biggest grocery store chain in the country, I'm figuring that's indicative of much of the nation.

☺ Vietnamese Chicken Salad

I tried making a really authentic Vietnamese Chicken Salad, and it was delicious—but it also took forever to make—including an hour and a half to poach a whole chicken! I was determined to streamline the process so you could enjoy this wonderful treat. Here it is.

> 1 pound (455 g) boneless, skinless chicken breast or precooked chicken breast slices
>
> 6 cups (540 g) bagged coleslaw mix
>
> 4 scallions
>
> 1 batch *Nuoc Cham* (see page 292)
>
> 1 ruby red grapefruit
>
> 2 tablespoons (16 g) sesame seeds
>
> 2 tablespoons (12 g) chopped fresh mint
>
> 2 tablespoons (2 g) chopped fresh cilantro

If you're starting with raw chicken breasts, you'll want to start cooking them first. I do mine for about 6 minutes in my electric tabletop grill, but you could sauté them, if you prefer. If you're sautéing them, you may want to take a minute to pound them thin so they cook through within our 15-minute time limit. If you're really in a hurry, feel free to use precooked chicken breast slices instead, although you'll pay a premium for them.

Put the bagged coleslaw mix in a bowl and slice the scallions into it. Make the *Nuoc Cham*—this is very quick to do—pour it over the cabbage, and toss well. Set aside.

Cut the grapefruit in half and loosen the sections by running the tip of a knife around each one.

Put the sesame seeds in a small, dry skillet and shake them over a high flame for about 2 minutes or until they start to jump around in the pan and make popping sounds. Turn off the burner and set the pan aside.

Okay, the chicken is ready now! If you're using unsliced breasts, put them on a cutting board and thinly slice them.

Now, toss the cabbage one more time to make sure the dressing is evenly distributed. Mound it on 4 serving plates. Top each serving with sliced chicken. Spoon 1/4 of the grapefruit sections around each portion. Scatter 1 tablespoon each of (6 g) chopped mint and (1 g) chopped cilantro over each serving (or easier yet, use kitchen shears to snip the herbs directly onto each serving), scatter 1/2 tablespoon of sesame seeds over each plate, and serve.

Yield: 4 generous servings, each with 18 grams of carbohydrates and 5 grams of fiber, for a total of 13 grams of usable carbs (virtually all of them from vegetables!) and 30 grams of protein.

✻ This has less than 250 calories, too!

⊕ Cajun Chicken Salad

Make the *Cajun Dressing* on page 300 first. Even with the two recipes to get through, you can do this in 15 minutes.

> 1/4 cup (28 g) chopped pecans (I bought mine already chopped.)
> 1 teaspoon butter
> 1 celery rib, diced
> 3 scallions, sliced, including the crisp part of the green shoot
> 1/2 green bell pepper, diced
> 1/4 cup (15 g) chopped fresh parsley
> 1 1/2 cups (210 g) diced chicken
> 1 medium tomato diced
> Cajun Dressing (See recipe on page 300.)

This is your basic chicken salad procedure, with one little addition. The first thing you need to do is chop your pecans and start them sautéing over medium-low heat in the butter. Then just cut everything up, throw it in a bowl, add the pecans (they'll take about five minutes to toast), add the dressing, and toss. It's easy-peasy. Not to mention that it's good.

Yield: 3 servings, each with 482 calories, 41 grams fat, 23 grams protein, 8 grams carbohydrate, 3 grams dietary fiber, and 5 grams usable carb.

⊕ Chicken-Almond Noodle Salad

Roughly a million years ago, when I was working at the *Chicago School of Massage Therapy*, I used to walk out to a local health food store and—being sure back then that whole grains were good for me—buy a chicken-almond salad with whole wheat noodles for lunch. It's been years, and I don't know how close this comes, but it's reminiscent of that salad. It's darned good in its own right, anyway.

1 package tofu shirataki, fettuccini width

3 tablespoons (21 g) slivered almonds

1/2 tablespoon coconut oil

2 tablespoons (28 g) mayonnaise

1 tablespoon (14 g) almond butter

6 drops Sriracha hot sauce

1/2 teaspoon grated ginger root

2 teaspoons soy sauce

1/2 cup (70 g) cooked chicken

2 scallions, sliced thin, including the crisp part of the green

Snip open the packet of tofu shirataki and pour into a strainer in the sink. Rinse well and use your kitchen shears to snip across them a couple of times since they're so long. If you want, you can put them to soak in a bowl of fresh water, but I didn't bother.

In a small, heavy skillet, over medium-low heat, start your almonds sautéing in your coconut oil.

Measure your mayo, almond butter, Sriracha sauce, ginger root, and soy sauce into a smallish dish and stir together. This is your dressing.

Go back and stir your almonds! In fact, stir them once in between measuring the dressing ingredients. You don't want them to burn. When they're just getting golden, take them off the heat.

Cut your chicken into 1/2-inch (1.3 cm) cubes. Slice your scallions.

Okay, time to assemble your salad. Dump the shirataki into a mixing bowl (drain them again first if you've been soaking them in water.) Add the chicken, scallions, and toasted almonds, then the dressing. Stir it all up and you're done!

Yield: 2 servings, each with 326 calories, 28 grams fat, 16 grams protein, 6 grams carbohydrate, 2 grams dietary fiber, and 4 grams usable carb.

Note: I used leftover roasted chicken; I always roast more than I need so I have cold chicken in the fridge for just such purposes. But you could, instead, throw a boneless, skinless chicken breast into your electric tabletop grill as you were starting; it would add a minute or two to your prep time, but then I finished with a couple of minutes to spare anyway. Or you could use packaged, precooked chicken breast strips.

I think ¼ cup (3 g) of chopped water chestnuts would be nice in this, but keep in mind they'll add 4 grams of usable carb per serving.

⊕ Border Town Chicken Salad

If you don't have any leftover cooked chicken around the house, feel free to use canned, chunk chicken. It's not the same, but it's still good. Or you could cut up purchased, precooked chicken breast slices.

2 cups (280 g) diced, cooked chicken

3 stalks celery, diced

3 tablespoons (19 g) chopped ripe olives

3 tablespoons (3 g) chopped cilantro

1 batch *Guacamole Dressing* (see page 298)

6 scallions, sliced

Just chop everything up, make the dressing, combine it all, and toss. You can serve this on a bed of lettuce, if you like, but I've been known to eat mine straight out of the mixing bowl.

Yield: 4 servings, each with 9 grams of carbohydrates and 3 grams of fiber, for a total of 6 grams of usable carbs and 24 grams of protein.

✻ This salad is healthy, offering 720 milligrams of potassium and meaningful doses of calcium, vitamin A, and folic acid.

⏱ Satay Salad

Satay are little skewers of chicken or meat served with peanut sauce. This salad is quicker and easier than satay, and it turns what is usually an appetizer into a meal. This is also good if you substitute turkey tenderloins for the chicken breast. The 15-minute time on this recipe assumes that you've got *Dana's Chicken Seasoning* on hand—which, if you eat a lot of poultry, you should!

> 18 ounces (510 g) boneless, skinless chicken breast
>
> Dana's Chicken Seasoning (see page 303)
>
> 1/3 cup (80 ml) rice vinegar
>
> 3 tablespoons (48 g) natural peanut butter
>
> 2 tablespoons (3 g) Splenda
>
> 2 tablespoons (28 ml) oil
>
> 3/4 teaspoon grated gingerroot
>
> 2 tablespoons (28 ml) toasted sesame oil
>
> 1 tablespoon (15 ml) soy sauce
>
> 3 tablespoons (27 g) chopped dry-roasted peanuts
>
> 6 cups (282 g) bagged romaine mix
>
> 1 cup (90 g) bagged coleslaw mix
>
> 6 tablespoons (6 g) chopped cilantro
>
> 3/4 cup (78 g) bean sprouts

Preheat your electric tabletop grill.

Sprinkle both sides of the chicken breasts with *Dana's Chicken Seasoning* and slap them on the grill. Cook for 5 to 6 minutes or until cooked through.

While the chicken's grilling, put the vinegar, peanut butter, Splenda, oil, gingerroot, sesame oil, and soy sauce in a blender and run it for 10 to 20 seconds, scraping down the sides if needed. This is your dressing. Chop the peanuts while it's blending.

Assemble the romaine mix, coleslaw mix, cilantro, and bean sprouts in a large salad bowl. Pour the dressing over it and toss thoroughly. Divide between 3 serving plates.

By now the chicken should be done. Pull it out of the grill and slice each breast into thin strips. Divide the chicken between the 3 salads. Top each serving with 1 tablespoon (9 g) of chopped peanuts, and serve.

Yield: 3 servings, each with 14 grams of carbohydrates and 5 grams of fiber, for a total of 9 grams of usable carbs and 48 grams of protein.

✻ You'll also get 880 milligrams of potassium in each serving!

☺ Aladdin Salad

I thought I was done with this chapter. Then I went to the Aladdin Restaurant in San Diego and had this fantastic salad. It was easy to duplicate and way too good to leave out! If you're ever in San Diego, I highly recommend that you go to the Aladdin, by the way. I was very disappointed not to get back there before I left for home.

> Salt and pepper
> 8 ounces (225 g) boneless, skinless chicken breast
> 8 cups (376 g) romaine, broken up
> 8 tablespoons (8 g) chopped fresh cilantro
> 1/4 cup (40 g) thinly sliced sweet red onion
> 1/3 cup (80 ml) bottled balsamic vinaigrette—I like Paul Newman's.
> 1/2 cup (75 g) crumbled feta
> 1/3 cup (41 g) shelled pistachios*
> 1 medium ripe tomato

* Look for these at Mediterranean or Middle Eastern groceries or at a health food store with a good bulk section.

Preheat your electric tabletop grill while you salt and pepper the chicken lightly. Throw it on the grill and set a timer for 6 minutes or so.

While the chicken's cooking, put the romaine, cilantro, and onion in a large salad bowl, pour on the dressing, and toss well. Pile this mixture on 2 serving plates. Scatter the feta and pistachios over the greens.

When the chicken is done, slice it into strips and divide it between the 2 salads. Slice the tomato into eighths, arrange 4 slices around each salad, and then serve.

Yield: 2 large servings, each with 18 grams of carbohydrates and 7 grams of fiber, for a total of 11 grams of usable carbs and 40 grams of protein.

⭐ You'll also get 1,333 milligrams of potassium and 320 milligrams of calcium!

☺ Lemon-Basil-Artichoke Turkey Salad

So there I was, with a whole bunch of lemons and a huge pile of fresh basil. What's a girl to do? I came up with this dish.

> 1/2 teaspoon chopped garlic
>
> 1/2 cup (120 ml) extra virgin olive oil
>
> 1/2 head cauliflower
>
> 1 small diced red onion
>
> 8 jarred pepperoncini peppers
>
> 12 ounces (340 g) canned artichoke hearts
>
> 1/2 cup (20 g) fresh basil
>
> 1/2 cup (30 g) chopped fresh parsley
>
> 3 cups (420 g) diced turkey
>
> 1 lemon
>
> 1/3 cup (45 g) pine nuts

Crush the garlic clove, put it in a measuring cup, and pour the olive oil over it. Let it sit.

Trim the leaves and the very bottom of the stem off your half of a cauliflower, whack it into big chunks, and run it through the shredding blade of your food processor. Put the resulting cauli-rice in a microwaveable casserole with a lid, add a couple of tablespoons (28 ml) of water, cover, and nuke on high for 6 minutes.

Don't bother wiping out your food processor, just swap the shredding blade for the S-blade. Halve and peel your onion, cut it in a few chunks, throw it in, and pulse to chop fairly fine. Dump into a big salad bowl and put the bowl back on the base. Add the pepperoncini (cut off the stem ends first), pulse once or twice, and then throw in the drained artichoke hearts and pulse a few more times to chop to a medium consistency. Dump all that in the salad bowl, too.

Somewhere in all this chopping, your microwave will beep. Take out the cauli-rice and uncover it to stop the cooking. Let it cool while you finish chopping.

You can chop your basil and parsley in the food processor too, if you like, but I find a kitchen shears easier. I measured the first time, but from here on out I'd probably just snip right into the bowl and eyeball my quantities.

Finally, cube your turkey. I used a big hunk of deli turkey breast, but this would be a great way to use up Thanksgiving leftovers. Cut it in 1/2 inch (1.3 cm) cubes and throw it in the bowl, too.

Drain your cauli-rice, add it to the salad, and stir it all up.

Dump in the garlicky olive oil and halve and squeeze the lemon over the top (pick out any seeds first!). Add the pine nuts, toss one final time, and serve.

Yield: 5 servings, each with 451 calories, 32 grams fat, 26 grams protein, 18 grams carbohydrate, 6 grams dietary fiber, and 12 grams usable carb.

⊕ Club Sandwich Salad

This is all the flavors you loved in a club sandwich in a filling salad. The limiting factor in this recipe is your microwave—I assume you have only one! There just wasn't quite enough time in fifteen minutes to nuke both the cauliflower and the bacon sequentially. That's why I've specified precooked bacon. If you don't mind your recipe taking a few minutes more, go ahead and microwave your own bacon; it's cheaper and fresher. This is a great make-ahead, by the way.

> 1/2 head cauliflower
> 2 cups (280 g) diced turkey—leftover, or deli turkey
> 1 romaine lettuce heart, cut crosswise in 1/2 inch (1.3 cm) strips (about 4 cups
>   [228 g] lettuce)
> 2 medium tomatoes
> 10 slices precooked bacon

2 tablespoons (28 ml) cider vinegar

2 tablespoons (28 ml) lemon juice

1 teaspoon spicy brown mustard

1/2 cup (115 g) mayonnaise

salt and pepper

Trim the leaves and the very bottom of the stem off your half of a cauliflower, whack it into chunks, and run it through the shredding blade of your food processor. Put the resulting cauli-rice into a microwaveable casserole with a lid, add a couple of tablespoons (28 ml) of water, and nuke on high for six minutes.

In the meantime, cube your turkey—I used deli turkey and had the guys at the deli slice it a full half-inch (1.3 cm) thick, which made for nice cubes. Throw it in a big salad bowl. Shred your romaine, dice your tomatoes, and throw them in too.

Somewhere in here your microwave will beep. Pull out your cauli-rice and uncover it to stop the cooking. Let it cool a few minutes so it won't cook your lettuce and tomatoes! It will cool faster if you drain it and stir it now and then.

Measure and whisk together your vinegar, lemon juice, mustard, and mayonnaise.

Use your kitchen shears to snip the bacon into the salad; cut it every 1/4 inch (6 mm) or so. Now add the cauli-rice, pour on the dressing, toss well, and serve.

Yield: 5 servings, each with 353 calories, 29 grams fat, 19 grams protein, 7 grams carbohydrate, 3 grams dietary fiber, and 4 grams usable carb.

⊕Warm Chicken Liver Salad

You will like this if you like chicken livers, and you won't like it if you don't. Mmmmm. Chicken livers…

6 large chicken livers

2 tablespoons (28 ml) olive oil

Salt or Vege-Sal and pepper

8 ounces (225 g) bagged mixed greens—European or Parisian blends are good.

1/2 ripe avocado

1-inch (2.5 cm) wedge of a large sweet red onion, sliced paper thin

1/3 cup (80 ml) bottled Dijon vinaigrette

Cut each chicken liver into 3 or 4 pieces. Spray a large, heavy skillet with nonstick cooking spray and put it over medium-high heat. Add the oil and the livers. Sauté the livers, turning them frequently, until juices run clear and no pink spots show on the outsides. (Take care not to overcook the livers! They get tough if you overcook them.) Turn off the burner when they're done and if you have an electric stove, remove the pan from the warm element. Salt and pepper lightly.

Pour the bagged greens into a big salad bowl. Use the tip of a spoon to scoop bits of avocado out of the shell and into the salad bowl. Add the sliced onion, pour the dressing over it all, and toss well. Divide the salad mixture between 2 plates.

Top each salad with half of the livers and serve.

Yield: 2 servings, each with 15 grams of carbohydrates and 6 grams of fiber, for a total of 9 grams of usable carbs and 21 grams of protein.

⁂ This recipe is truly healthy. It gives you 892 milligrams of potassium and well over your daily requirement for vitamin A, vitamin C, vitamin B2, vitamin B12, and folacin, not to mention half of your daily requirement for niacin, B6, and iron, and good doses of calcium, zinc, and B1. Indeed, I toyed with the idea of calling this *Big Pile of Nutrition Salad*. It's got to be the most nutritious recipe in the book.

⊕ Chicken Liver Salad with Warm Bacon Dressing

I love chicken livers, and despite dire pronouncements about it being *the filter of the body*, liver is about the most nutritious food there is. This is a snap to double, by the way, should you have another liver-lover in the house.

> 2 bacon slices
>
> 2 tablespoons (16 g) coconut flour
>
> 1/4 teaspoon salt or Vege-Sal
>
> 1/4 teaspoon pepper
>
> 1/4 teaspoon ground allspice
>
> 3 chicken livers

1/2 teaspoon chopped garlic

1 tablespoon bacon grease (15 g) or olive oil (15 ml)

3 tablespoons (45 ml) sherry vinegar

1/8 medium red onion, sliced paper-thin

3 cups (170 g) mixed lettuce

1 cup (20 g) arugula

Put a biggish heavy skillet over medium heat and use your kitchen shears to snip the bacon into it. You want it to wind up in bacon bits. Let the bacon fry.

In a cereal bowl, mix together the coconut flour, salt, pepper, and allspice. Go stir your bacon.

Use that same kitchen shears to snip each liver into 2 to 3 pieces, right into the seasoned coconut flour. Toss them around until they're coated.

Put your lettuce and arugula in a big bowl and slice your onion and have it standing by.

By now your bacon should be crisp. Fish it out with a slotted spatula (slotted because you want the grease to stay in the pan) and throw in your floured chicken liver chunks. Fry them quickly until they're just browned all over. The juice should still be running pink. Fish those out and put them on the plate with the bacon bits.

Throw the garlic, the extra bacon grease or olive oil, and the vinegar in the skillet and boil it for a second or two, scraping up all the yummy browned bits. Pour this over the lettuce and toss. Top with the red onion, liver, and bacon bits, and eat.

By the way, you can pile your greens on a plate if you want, but I ate mine out of the salad bowl I tossed them in. It's easier.

Yield: 1 serving, with 462 calories, 26 grams fat, 26 grams protein, 31 grams carbohydrate, 14 grams dietary fiber, and 17 grams usable carb.

☉ Warm Chicken Liver and Artichoke Salad

I adapted this from a recipe that wanted you to start by cooking artichokes and trimming out their hearts, then marinating them. Starting with marinated artichoke hearts seemed a lot simpler and it certainly tastes good.

  3 tablespoons (45 ml) olive oil, divided

  1 tablespoon (15 ml) sherry vinegar

  2 drops orange extract

  1/4 teaspoon spicy brown or Dijon mustard

  1 pinch Splenda

  1/8 medium onion

  1/4 teaspoon chopped garlic

  3/4 cup (225 g) marinated artichoke hearts, quartered—Buy them that way!

  4 chicken livers

  3 cups (90 g) fresh baby spinach

  1/8 small red onion, sliced paper-thin

  salt and pepper

Put the 2 tablespoons (28 ml) of the olive oil, plus the vinegar, orange extract, mustard, Splenda, onion, and garlic in your blender or food processor and run until smooth and creamy. Put this by the stove.

Drain and measure the artichoke hearts. Snip the livers into two or three chunks each, depending on size, and dust them with salt and pepper. Put your spinach on a plate, slice the onion, and put it on top.

Okay, it's cooking time: Give a medium-sized heavy skillet a shot of nonstick cooking spray and put it over medium heat. Add the last tablespoon (15 ml) of olive oil and slosh it around to coat. When it's hot, throw in the livers and sauté until the surfaces are *seized* and the blood stops running but take care not to overcook. They should still be pink inside. Add the artichoke hearts and dressing and stir until everything's just warm through, scraping up the tasty brown bits from the bottom of the skillet. Pile the livers and artichokes on the spinach and eat.

Yield: 1 to 2 servings, assuming 1, it will have 714 calories, 55 grams fat, 32 grams protein, 24 grams carbohydrate, 9 grams dietary fiber, and 15 grams usable carb.

⊕ Ham-Pecan Salad with Apricot Dressing

Always read the labels and buy the lowest-sugar ham you can find—they vary quite a lot in carbohydrate content. This recipe assumes ham with 1 gram per 3 ounce (85 g) serving.

5 ounces (140 g) cooked ham, diced

1 stalk celery, diced

2 tablespoons (20 g) diced red onion

1/4 cup (28 g) chopped pecans

2 tablespoons (28 g) mayonnaise

2 teaspoons low-sugar apricot preserves

1 teaspoon spicy brown or Dijon mustard

1/4 teaspoon soy sauce

Mix together the ham, celery, onion, and pecans in a mixing bowl. Combine the mayonnaise, preserves, mustard, and soy sauce and pour this over the ham mixture. Mix well and serve. This is really nice on a bed of lettuce.

Yield: 1 serving, with 15 grams of carbohydrates and 4 grams of fiber, for a total of 11 grams of usable carbs and 29 grams of protein.

⊕ Buttery Ham-Pineapple-Pea Salad

You know how it is with ham: The whole family loves it until they see the leftovers *again*. Here's a great way to turn leftover ham into a whole new dish. If you don't have any leftover ham, you can buy a chunk of precooked ham at the grocery store.

1/2 head cauliflower

1 small red onion

3/4 cup (124 g) pineapple chunks, fresh or canned in juice

1 cup (130 g) frozen peas

8 ounces (225 g) cooked ham

2 tablespoons (28 g) butter

2 tablespoons (28 g) DaVinci sugar-free pineapple syrup

2 tablespoons (28 ml) rice vinegar or white wine vinegar

1 tablespoon (15 ml) olive oil

1 tablespoon (15 ml) lemon or lime juice

2 tablespoons (22 g) spicy brown or Dijon mustard

salt and pepper to taste

Run the cauliflower through the shredding blade of your food processor. Put the resulting cauli-rice in a microwaveable casserole with a lid, add a couple of table-spoons (28 ml) of water, cover, and nuke on high for 6 minutes.

While that's happening, swap out the shredding blade for the S-blade. Peel your onion, whack it into chunks, and throw it in. Pulse until it's chopped to a medium consistency. Dump this in a big mixing bowl.

Put the food processor bowl back on the base and throw in the pineapple. Pulse until it's a medium-coarse consistency—you still want recognizable chunks of pine-apple; you just want them to distribute through the salad. Dump this in the mixing bowl as well.

Measure the peas and throw them in, too. No need to thaw them—the hot cauli-flower will do that, and the peas will help cool the salad.

Cut your ham in small cubes. (Or you could chop it in the food processor, but I like cubes somewhere between 1/4 inch and 1/2 inch [6 to 13 mm].) Add them to the bowl.

Somewhere in here the microwave will beep. Haul out your cauli-rice, uncover it, and drain it very well. Add it to the mixing bowl and throw the butter on top of it so it will melt. Toss the whole thing, making sure the butter gets distributed well.

Now mix together the pineapple syrup, vinegar, oil, lemon or lime juice, and mustard. Pour over the salad and toss again. Salt and pepper to taste and serve.

Yield: 4 servings, each with 253 calories, 16 grams fat, 13 grams protein, 16 grams carbohydrate, 3 grams dietary fiber, and 13 grams usable carb.

Note: That pineapple syrup is kind of handy to have around. I mix it half-and-half with soy sauce and add a little grated ginger root and garlic to get a quick teriyaki sauce. It's worth stocking.

⊕ Italian Roast Beef Salad

What a great meal, all from deli roast beef! Feel free to use leftover steak in this instead, should you happen to have any.

- 2 quarts (570 g) bagged European or Italian blend greens
- ¼ cup (40 g) thinly sliced sweet red onion
- ¼ medium green pepper, sliced into small strips
- 3 tablespoons (45 ml) extra virgin olive oil
- ½ teaspoon minced garlic or 1 clove garlic, crushed
- 1 ½ tablespoons (23 ml) balsamic vinegar
- ½ teaspoon spicy brown or Dijon mustard
- ¼ cup (30 g) crumbled Gorgonzola cheese
- 4 ounces (115 g) sliced deli roast beef
- 2 tablespoons (18 g) toasted pine nuts

Place the greens, onion, and green pepper in a large salad bowl. Combine the oil and garlic, pour over the salad, and toss well. Stir together the balsamic vinegar and mustard and set them aside.

Crumble the Gorgonzola (if you didn't buy it precrumbled) and add it to the salad. Slice the roast beef into strips and throw it in there, too. Pour the balsamic vinegar mixture over the whole thing and toss very well. Pile onto 2 serving plates, top each with a tablespoon (9 g) of pine nuts, and serve.

Yield: 2 servings, each with 19 grams of carbohydrates and 9 grams of fiber, for a total of 10 grams of usable carbs and 27 grams of protein.

✳ You'll also get 1,153 milligrams of potassium and 247 milligrams of calcium, plus almost three times your daily requirements of vitamins C and A, and 100 percent of your daily requirement of folacin.

. . . .

Note: Gorgonzola is the Italian version of blue cheese, a bit milder and creamier than most blue cheeses. If you can't find it, substitute any blue cheese you like.

. . . .

☺Hamburger Salad with Sundried Tomato and Chipotle Dressing

Yes, it's a main dish salad with a whole hamburger plunked on top. And a fine thing it is, too.

3 slices bacon

12 ounces (340 g) ground chuck

1/2 cup (115 g) mayonnaise

5 sun-dried tomato halves

1 chipotle chile canned in adobo

1/2 teaspoon chopped garlic

1 tablespoon (15 ml) cider vinegar

2 tablespoons (28 ml) olive oil

1 bag (10 ounces, or 280 g) Italian blend lettuce

3 cups (60 g) arugula

1/4 red onion

Start preheating your electric tabletop grill.

Lay your bacon on a microwave bacon rack or in a Pyrex pie plate and nuke on high for 4 to 6 minutes or until crisp.

Make three hamburger patties and set them by the grill, ready to go.

Put the mayonnaise in your food processor with the S-blade in place. Snip your tomato halves into your food processor (you can chop them instead, but I find snipping them with my kitchen shears quicker and easier.) Add the chipotle and a teaspoon of the adobo sauce, the garlic, the vinegar, and the olive oil. Turn on the processor!

By now your grill is hot. Throw in the hamburgers and set a timer for 4 to 5 minutes.

Go turn off the food processor; you should have dressing.

Okay, we're getting to the finish line: Dump the lettuce and arugula into a big salad bowl. Pour on most of the dressing, reserving a few spoonfuls to top the burgers. Toss and toss and toss until everything is coated. Pile the salad on three plates.

Slice your onion quarter paper thin and distribute it between the three plates. Crumble a slice of bacon over each salad. When the burgers are done, put one on each salad, top with the reserved dressing, and serve.

Yield: 3 servings, each with 720 calories, 67 grams fat, 25 grams protein, 9 grams carbohydrate, 3 grams dietary fiber, and 6 grams total carb.

chapter eight

15~Minute Skillet Suppers

One-dish skillet meals are quick, versatile, and—since they generally contain both your protein and your vegetable—they eliminate the need to cook anything else. Furthermore, there's only one pan to wash!

Some of these "skillet suppers" can also be cooked in a wok. Use whatever you have.

☉ Asian Pork and Cabbage

I know of few dishes that offer so much flavor for so little work.

> 1 pound (455 g) boneless pork loin
>
> 1/2 head cabbage
>
> 1 small onion
>
> Canola or peanut oil for stir-frying
>
> 1 tablespoon (15 g) black bean sauce
>
> 1 to 2 tablespoons (16 to 32 g) chili garlic paste

Slice the pork loin as thin as you possibly can—this is easier if the pork is partially frozen. Slice the cabbage about 1/2-inch (1.3 cm) thick, and cut across it a few times. Thinly slice the onion.

In a wok or large skillet, heat 3 to 4 tablespoons (45 to 60 ml) of oil over highest heat. As soon as it's hot, add the pork and stir-fry for 3 to 5 minutes. Add the cabbage and the onion and continue stir-frying until the cabbage and onion are just tender-crisp. Stir in the black bean sauce and the chili garlic paste and serve.

Yield: 3 servings, each with 6 grams of carbohydrates and 1 gram of fiber, for a total of 5 grams of usable carbs and 32 grams of protein.

> **Note:** Find Black Bean Sauce, an Asian condiment, in Asian or International grocery stores or in the Asian section of larger grocery stores. I actually bought mine in the International aisle of Bloomingfoods, my beloved health food store. This has some sugar in it, but the amount of flavor it offers for the few carbs it adds is well worth it, to my mind. It keeps well in the fridge, so don't think you have to use it all up quickly.

⊕ Balsamic Lamb Skillet

This dish is rich, different, and good!

> 1 pound (455 g) lamb leg or shoulder, thinly sliced and cut into strips
>
> 1/2 teaspoon minced garlic or 1 clove garlic, crushed
>
> 1/2 medium onion, sliced
>
> 1/4 cup (60 ml) olive oil
>
> 1/2 red bell pepper, sliced into small strips
>
> 1 bag (16 ounces, or 455 g) triple-washed fresh spinach
>
> 1/4 cup (60 ml) balsamic vinegar
>
> Salt and pepper
>
> Guar or xanthan
>
> 4 tablespoons (36 g) toasted pine nuts

Over high heat, start sautéing the lamb, garlic, and onion in the olive oil. When the pinkness has faded from the lamb, add the red bell pepper and stir that in, too.

When the lamb is cooked through and the onion is limp, add the spinach. You may have to add it in two or three batches to keep it from overwhelming your skillet, but it wilts quite quickly. Stir until the spinach is just barely limp. Don't overcook!

Stir in the balsamic vinegar, salt and pepper to taste (I like plenty of pepper in this), and thicken the pan juices with a sprinkle of guar or xanthan, if desired. Serve and top each serving with a tablespoon (9 g) of toasted pine nuts.

Yield: 4 servings, each with 9 grams of carbohydrates and 4 grams of fiber, for a total of 5 grams of usable carbs and 20 grams of protein.

⊕ Curried Lamb with Peas

This is not authentically Indian or authentically anything, I'm guessing, but it's fast and good. You could make this with ground beef instead, but the lamb is best and a nice change.

1 cup (130 g) frozen peas

1 pound (455 g) ground lamb

1/2 medium onion

1 1/2 teaspoons chopped garlic

1 1/2 tablespoons (9 g) curry powder

1/2 teaspoon ground cinnamon

1 tablespoon (8 g) grated gingerroot

1/2 teaspoon salt or to taste

Give your big, heavy skillet a squirt of nonstick cooking spray and put it over a medium burner to heat. Put your peas, still frozen, in a microwaveable bowl, add a tablespoon (15 ml) or so of water, cover (I use a saucer), and nuke on high for 3 to 4 minutes.

While that's happening, throw your lamb in your hot skillet and start browning and crumbling it. When it's broken up and starting to cook a little, put a tilted lid on it to hold the heat in.

Whack your half an onion into a few chunks and throw it in your food processor. Pulse to chop. When it's a medium texture, go dump it in with the lamb and stir everything up. Re-cover the lamb while you crush your garlic and then throw that in, too. Stir in the spices.

By now, your peas are cooked! Dump those in the skillet, too, and stir them in. Keep cooking and stirring until the lamb and onion are cooked through and serve.

Yield: 3 servings, each with 488 calories, 36 grams fat, 28 grams protein, 12 grams carbohydrate, 4 grams dietary fiber, and 8 grams usable carb.

⊙ Chicken Skillet Alfredo

Who doesn't love Alfredo sauce?

> 1 1/2 pounds (680 g) boneless, skinless chicken breast
>
> 1/2 medium onion
>
> 3 tablespoons (45 ml) olive oil
>
> 1 bag (16 ounces, or 455 g) frozen mixed cauliflower and broccoli or 1/2 pound
> (225 g) frozen broccoli florets and 1/2 pound (225 g) frozen cauliflowerets
>
> 1 cup (250 ml) jarred Alfredo sauce
>
> Parmesan cheese (optional)

Cut the chicken into 1-inch (2.5 cm) cubes and slice your onion. Sauté the chicken and onion in the olive oil over medium heat.

While the chicken and onion are cooking, put the cauliflower and broccoli in a microwaveable casserole. Add a tablespoon or two (15 to 28 ml) of water, cover, and nuke it on High for 7 minutes. Go back and stir the chicken and onion while the veggies are nuking.

When the microwave goes "ding," check to see if the veggies are tender but not mushy. If they need a couple more minutes, give it to them. When the broccoli and cauliflower are done, drain them and add them to the skillet. Stir in the Alfredo sauce, heat through, and serve. Pass a little Parmesan to sprinkle on top, if you like.

Yield: 5 servings, each with 8 grams of carbohydrates and 3 grams of fiber, for a total of 5 grams of usable carbs and 35 grams of protein.

⊕ Chicken Skillet Roma

1 1/2 pounds (680 g) boneless, skinless chicken breast, cut into 1-inch (2.5 cm) cubes

1/2 green pepper, cut into small strips

1 small onion, sliced

2 cloves garlic, crushed, or 1 teaspoon minced garlic

3 tablespoons (45 ml) olive oil

1 can (2 1/4 ounces, or 70 g) can sliced ripe olives, drained

1 cup (245 g) no-sugar-added spaghetti sauce

1/4 cup (25 g) grated Parmesan cheese

Sauté the chicken, pepper, onion, and garlic in the olive oil over medium-high heat. When all the pink is gone from the chicken, stir in the olives and spaghetti sauce, bring it to a simmer, and let it cook for just another minute. Serve with the Parmesan cheese on top.

Yield: 5 servings, each with 8 grams of carbohydrates and 2 grams of fiber, for a total of 6 grams of usable carbs and 33 grams of protein.

⊕ Italian Sausage with Onions and Peppers

Mmmmmmm! It's like revisiting my childhood in the New York City area!

> 1 1/4 to 1 1/2 pounds (570 to 680 g) Italian sausage links, hot or mild
>
> 1/4 cup (60 ml) olive oil
>
> 1 1/2 large green peppers
>
> 1 large onion
>
> 1 clove garlic

Slice the sausage diagonally into 1/2-inch (1.3 cm) pieces and sauté it in the olive oil over medium-high heat. Meanwhile, slice the peppers into medium-size strips and slice the onion about 1/4 inch (6 mm) thick. When the sausage is about half done, stir in the peppers, onion, and garlic. Cook until the sausage is well done and the onion is limp and translucent. Serve.

Yield: 4 servings, each with 7 grams of carbohydrates and 1 gram of fiber, for a total of 6 grams of usable carbs and 21 grams of protein.

⊕ Italian Sausage with Onions, Peppers, Tomato Sauce, and Cheese

Make *the Italian Sausage with Onions and Peppers* as described above. When it's done, stir in the following:

> 1 cup (245 g) no-sugar-added spaghetti sauce

Then top with the following:

> 1 cup (115 g) shredded mozzarella cheese

Cover the skillet for a couple of minutes to let the sauce heat through and the cheese melt. Serve.

Yield: 4 servings, each with 12 grams of carbohydrates and 3 grams of fiber, for a total of 9 grams of usable carbs and 28 grams of protein.

Note: One of the lowest carbohydrate nationally distributed spaghetti sauces is Hunt's Original Style No Sugar Added. (They also make an Original Style with sugar, so read the label!) Each 1/2-cup (123 g) serving contains 9 grams of carbohydrates and 3 grams of fiber, for a total of 6 grams of usable carbs. I really like this stuff!

⊕ New-Fangled Farm Fry

In Peg Bracken's classic cookbook, *The I Hate To Cook Book*, there was a recipe for eggs cooked with potatoes, onions, and cheese, called "Old Fashioned Farm Fry." Here's my low-carb, twenty-first century version.

4 slices bacon

1 cup (100 g) cauliflowerets, chopped into 1/2-inch (1.5 cm) pieces

1 cup (150 g) diced turnip, chopped into 1/2-inch (1.5 cm) pieces

1/2 cup (80 g) diced onion

4 eggs

1/2 cup (58 g) shredded cheddar cheese

Salt and pepper

Chop the bacon up into smallish bits—kitchen shears are good for this. Start the bacon cooking in a big skillet. Combine the cauliflowerets and turnip in a microwaveable dish, add a couple of tablespoons (28 ml) of water, cover, and microwave on High for 7 minutes.

Drain the vegetables when they're done. Drain all but a few tablespoons (45 to 60 ml) of fat off the bacon, and add the cauliflower, turnip, and onion to the skillet. Sauté until the onion is translucent. Scramble the eggs with a fork, pour them into the skillet, sprinkle the cheese over the whole thing, and stir until the eggs are set. Salt and pepper to taste and serve.

Yield: 2 servings, each with 12 grams of carbohydrates and 3 grams of fiber, for a total of 9 grams of usable carbs and 24 grams of protein.

⊕ Shrimp and Mushroom Sauté

This is quick and easy enough for the family, yet it's impressive enough for company!

2 tablespoons (28 ml) olive oil

2 tablespoons (28 g) butter

8 ounces (225 g) sliced mushrooms

1/2 medium onion

1 pound (455 g) cleaned, shelled shrimp

1/2 teaspoon minced garlic or 1 clove garlic, crushed

1 tablespoon (15 ml) lemon juice

1 tablespoon (15 ml) dry white wine

Heat the olive oil and butter together in a heavy skillet over medium-high heat. Add the mushrooms and onion and sauté until the vegetables start to soften. Add the shrimp and cook until they're pink all over and the onion is translucent. Stir in the garlic, lemon juice, and wine, cook for just another minute or two, and then serve.

Yield: 3 servings, each with 7 grams of carbohydrates and 1 gram of fiber, for a total of 6 grams of usable carbs and 32 grams of protein.

⊕ Smoked Sausage and Sprouts

This is a speeded-up version of a dish in *500 Low-Carb Recipes*—just cut things into smaller bits, and they cook faster!

> 1 pound (455 g) smoked sausage
>
> 2 tablespoons (28 g) butter
>
> 1 pound (455 g) brussels sprouts
>
> 1/4 cup (40 g) diced onion

Slice the smoked sausage diagonally into 1/2-inch thick (1.3 cm) pieces. Melt the butter in a heavy skillet over medium-high heat and start cooking the sausage in it. Meanwhile, run the brussels sprouts through the slicing blade of your food processor. Add the brussels sprouts and onion to the skillet and continue to cook everything, stirring occasionally, until the brussels sprouts are wilted and the sausage is hot right through. Serve.

Yield: 4 servings, each with 12 grams of carbohydrates and 4 grams of fiber, for a total of 8 grams of usable carbs (less if you choose very low-carb smoked sausage) and 19 grams of protein.

Note: Smoked sausage varies a lot in carb count. Read your labels carefully!

☉ Sour Cream Ham Supper

Another updated, decarbed recipe from Peg Bracken's classic, *The I Hate To Cook Book*.

    1/2 head cauliflower

    1/2 medium onion, diced

    2 cups (300 g) cooked ham, cut into strips

    8 ounces (225 g) sliced mushrooms

    2 tablespoons (28 g) butter

    1/2 cup (115 g) sour cream

Run the cauliflower through the shredding blade of your food processor. Put it in a microwaveable casserole, add a couple of tablespoons (28 ml) of water, cover, and nuke on High for 6 to 7 minutes.

While the cauliflower is cooking, dice the onion and cut the ham into smallish strips. Melt the butter in a large, heavy skillet over medium heat and sauté the onion, ham, and mushrooms in it, stirring frequently. When the onion is limp and translucent, turn the burner to low and stir in the sour cream. Heat through but don't let it come to a boil or the sour cream will "crack."

Drain the cauliflower, divide it between 3 plates, and spoon the ham mixture over it.

Yield: 3 servings, each with 9 grams of carbohydrates and 1 gram of fiber, for a total of 8 grams of usable carbs and 19 grams of protein.

☉ Unstuffed Cabbage

Stuffed cabbage is a perennial favorite, but there's no way to stuff all those leaves and get 'em cooked in 15 minutes! Here's a recipe that gives you all the flavor of stuffed cabbage at breakneck speed. Do use very lean ground beef for this recipe—it saves you the time needed to drain off the grease.

> 1 1/2 pounds (680 g) ground round or other very lean ground beef
>
> 1 medium onion, chopped
>
> 1 teaspoon minced garlic or 2 cloves garlic, crushed
>
> 1/2 head cabbage, coarsely chopped
>
> 1 can (8 ounces, or 225 g) tomato sauce
>
> 2 tablespoons (28 ml) lemon juice
>
> 1/2 teaspoon pepper
>
> 1/2 teaspoon ground nutmeg
>
> 1/2 teaspoon ground cinnamon
>
> 1 teaspoon salt

Start the ground beef cooking in a heavy skillet over high heat; spread it out to cover the bottom of the pan so it cooks quicker.

While the ground beef is browning, chop the onion and crush the garlic. Plunk them in the pan with the ground beef and stir it up using a spatula to turn it over and break it up so that it cooks evenly. Cover the pan and let it continue cooking.

Meanwhile, chop the cabbage coarsely. Stir this into the beef mixture a bit at a time—it will come close to overwhelming your skillet, unless yours is bigger than mine. Again, take care to turn everything over to keep it cooking evenly. Re-cover the pan.

Continue to stir the meat mixture to keep it cooking evenly, covering in between stirrings. When the cabbage is starting to wilt, stir in the tomato sauce, lemon juice, pepper, nutmeg, cinnamon, and salt. Re-cover, let the whole thing simmer for 5 minutes, and then serve.

Yield: 5 servings, each with 7 grams of carbohydrates and 2 grams of fiber, for a total of 5 grams of usable carbs and 25 grams of protein.

⊕ Spanish "Rice"

Okay, this isn't really Spanish. It's not even authentically Mexican. And of course it's not rice. But it is passingly like the "Spanish Rice" my mom used to throw together to make a quick, one-dish meal out of hamburger! Feel free to used canned, diced tomatoes without the chilies if you don't like spicy food, although this is really quite mild.

1 pound (455 g) ground round or other very lean ground beef

1 to 2 tablespoons (15 to 28 ml) oil

1/2 head cauliflower

1/2 green pepper, chopped

1/2 medium onion, chopped

1 teaspoon minced garlic

1 can (14.5 ounces, or 410 g) diced tomatoes with green chilies

1/2 teaspoon ground cumin

1 teaspoon Worcestershire sauce

1/4 cup (60 ml) water

Salt and pepper

Start browning the beef in the oil over medium-high heat. Meanwhile, run the cauliflower through the shredding blade of your food processor. Put the cauliflower in a microwavable casserole, add a tablespoon or two (15 to 28 ml) of water, cover, and microwave on High for just 5 minutes.

Go back to the beef and start breaking it up. When you've got just a little fat in the pan, add the pepper and onion and sauté them, too. When all the pink is gone from the meat, add the garlic, tomatoes, cumin, Worcestershire sauce, and water, and bring the whole thing to a simmer. Stir in the cauliflower "rice," cover, and let the whole thing simmer for 3 to 5 minutes. Salt and pepper to taste and serve.

Yield: 4 or 5 servings. Assuming 4 servings, each will have 7 grams of carbohydrates and 1 gram of fiber, for a total of 6 grams of usable carbs and 23 grams of protein.

☉ Fried "Rice"

This recipe is infinitely variable, and it is particularly good for using up any sort of leftover meat you have hanging about. If you don't have any leftovers, feel free to use cooked ham you bought at the grocery store, a can or two of chunk chicken or salad shrimp, or what-have-you.

> 1/2 head cauliflower
> Oil
> 2 eggs, beaten
> 1 1/2 cups (340 g) diced or shredded leftover cooked meat, canned meat, or seafood
> 1 cup (225 g) vegetables*
> 8 to 10 scallions, sliced, including the crisp part of the green
> 2 tablespoons (28 ml) soy sauce
> 1/2 teaspoon Splenda

* Use snow peas (chopped into 1-inch [2.5 cm] pieces), bean sprouts, shredded cabbage, water chestnuts, bamboo shoots—whatever is on hand and sounds good. One or two kinds are better than a mish-mash of half a dozen.

Run the cauliflower through the shredding blade of your food processor. Put the cauliflower in a microwaveable casserole, add a tablespoon or two (15 to 28 ml) of water, cover, and microwave on High for 5 minutes.

Spray a medium-size skillet with nonstick cooking spray and place over medium heat. Add a tablespoon (15 ml) of oil to coat the bottom of the skillet. Pour in the eggs and cover for a minute or so. Let the eggs cook in a flat sheet on the bottom of the skillet. When cooked through, remove and set aside.

Remove the cauliflower from the microwave and drain it. Put a few tablespoons (45 to 60 ml) of oil in a large, heavy skillet or wok, Stir in the meat, vegetables, and scallions. Cook, stirring occasionally, until the veggies are tender-crisp. Add the cauliflower rice and stir to blend. Shred the sheet of eggs and stir in the egg strips. Combine the soy sauce with the Splenda and stir into the fried "rice."

Yield: 2 or 3 servings. Obviously, the carb count on this will vary a little with what ingredients you use. However, assuming that you use the remains of a rotisserie chicken and half bean sprouts, half snow peas for your vegetables, and that you make 3 servings, each will have 8 grams of carbohydrates and 2 grams of fiber, for a total of 6 grams of usable carbs and 27 grams of protein.

☉ Chicken Chop Suey

4 tablespoons (60 ml) soy sauce

2 teaspoons Splenda

1 1/2 pounds (680 g) boneless, skinless chicken breast

8 to 10 scallions

3 to 4 tablespoons (45 to 60 ml) oil—peanut or canola is best

3 cups (312 g) bean sprouts

3 teaspoons (45 ml) toasted sesame oil

1/2 teaspoon chicken bouillon granules

Guar or xanthan

Mix together the soy sauce and Splenda in a little dish and set aside.

Slice the chicken breast into strips as thin as possible (this is easier to do if it's half-frozen). Cut the scallions into pieces about 1/2-inch (1.3 cm) long, using all the crisp part of the green.

Assemble all the ingredients by the stove. Place a wok or heavy skillet over highest heat and add the oil. Give it 30 seconds to 1 minute to heat and then add the chicken. Stir-fry for 4 to 5 minutes or until the pink is gone. Add the scallions and bean sprouts and stir-fry for another 1 to 2 minutes. Add the soy sauce mixture, sesame oil, bouillon granules, and a sprinkle of guar or xanthan to thicken the juices. Stir-fry for just another minute and then serve.

Yield: 4 or 5 servings. Assuming 4 servings, each will have 9 grams of carbohydrates and 3 grams of fiber, for a total of 6 grams of usable carbs and 42 grams of protein.

⊕ Hamburger Chop Suey

1 pound (455 g) ground round or other very lean ground beef

2 tablespoons (28 ml) oil

1 medium onion, sliced

2 cups (140 g) sliced mushrooms

2 stalks celery, thinly sliced on the diagonal

1/2 green pepper, diced

1/2 teaspoon minced garlic or 1 clove garlic, crushed

2 cups (208 g) bean sprouts

1/3 cup (80 ml) soy sauce

1/2 teaspoon liquid beef bouillon concentrate

In a wok or large skillet over high heat, start browning the beef in oil and breaking it up. When it's about halfway browned, add the onion, mushrooms, celery, green pepper, and garlic. Continue breaking up the meat while stir-frying the vegetables. When all the pink is gone from the beef and the veggies are almost tender-crisp, add the bean sprouts, soy sauce, and beef bouillon concentrate. Continue stir-frying until the bean sprouts are just barely starting to wilt and then serve.

Yield: 4 servings, each with 8 grams of carbohydrates and 2 grams of fiber, for a total of 6 grams of usable carbs and 24 grams of protein.

⊕ Crack Slaw

There are about a million versions of this recipe kicking around the internet, some low carb, some full of ramen noodles. It's filling, cheap, quick, and good. Feel free to play around with this—add green or red peppers, celery, or bean sprouts, whatever appeals. The essential parts are the ground beef, shredded cabbage, soy sauce, and sesame oil.

> 1 pound (455 g) ground chuck
>
> 8 ounces (225 g) sliced mushrooms
>
> 1 packet tofu shirataki, spaghetti or angel hair width
>
> 3 cups (210 g) bagged coleslaw mix
>
> 4 tablespoons (60 ml) soy sauce
>
> 2 tablespoons (28 ml) dark sesame oil
>
> 2 teaspoons chopped garlic
>
> 3 teaspoons (1.5 g) Splenda, or its equivalent in sweetness
>
> 10 scallions, sliced
>
> Sriracha hot sauce to taste

Put your biggest skillet over medium-high heat and start the ground chuck browning. As soon as a little fat starts to cook out of it, dump in the sliced mushrooms (you bought them sliced, right?) and break them up some more with the edge of your spatula. Stir and cover with that tilted lid.

Snip open your packet of shirataki and dump them in a strainer. Rinse and snip them a few times. Go back and stir your meat! Re-cover, of course.

When the beef is about 3/4 browned, stir in the cabbage, the drained shirataki, soy sauce, sesame oil, garlic, and Splenda. Re-cover with that tilted lid.

Slice up your scallions. Stir the meat again!

When the beef is done and the mushrooms are softened, stir in the scallions and hot sauce and serve.

Yield: 4 servings, each with 412 calories, 31 grams fat, 24 grams protein, 11 grams carbohydrate, 3 grams dietary fiber, and 8 grams usable carb.

⊕ Casual Chan's Special

In my first cookbook, *500 Low-Carb Recipes*, I included a recipe called *Joe*, involving hamburger, spinach, and eggs. The original name of that recipe—found in many versions, in many places—was Joe's Special or Casual Joe's Special. This is a similar recipe with a slight Asian accent, hence the name. This is easy to double, by the way.

1/2 pound (225 g) ground round or other very lean ground beef

1 tablespoon (15 ml) oil

2 scallions, sliced

1 cup (104 g) bean sprouts

2 eggs

1/2 teaspoon soy sauce

Salt and pepper

Start browning the beef in the oil in a large, heavy skillet over medium-high heat. While it's browning, you can slice the scallions, measure the bean sprouts, and whisk up the eggs together with the soy sauce.

Go back to the stove and start breaking up the beef. When it's crumbled and there's no pink left, add the scallions and sprouts. Stir for a minute or two—just long enough for the veggies to get hot through, but not long enough for the bean sprouts to get limp and soggy. Add the eggs and soy sauce and scramble until set. Salt and pepper to taste and serve.

Yield: 2 servings, each with 5 grams of carbohydrates and 1 gram of fiber, for a total of 4 grams of usable carbs and 29 grams of protein.

⊕ Beef and Artichoke Skillet

This is both different and good. Because quite a lot of the carbs in artichokes are in the form of inulin, a very low-impact carb, this is even easier on your blood sugar than the carb count would suggest.

    8 slices bacon

    1 1/2 pounds (680 g) boneless beef—sirloin or chuck are fine

    1/2 medium onion, thinly sliced

    2 tablespoons (28 ml) olive oil

    1/4 cup (60 ml) cider vinegar

    1 tablespoon Splenda

    1/2 teaspoon pepper

    1/2 teaspoon minced garlic or 1 clove garlic, crushed

    1 can (14 ounces, or 390 g) quartered artichoke hearts, drained

Lay the bacon on a microwave bacon rack or in a glass pie plate. Microwave on High for 8 minutes.

While the bacon is cooking, slice the beef as thinly as you can and then cut across the strips a couple of times, so they're no more than 2- to 3-inches long (5 to 7.5 cm). (This is easiest if the meat is partly frozen.) Slice up the onion now, too.

Heat the oil in a large, heavy skillet over high heat and start stir-frying the beef and onion. When the pink is gone from the beef, add the vinegar, Splenda, pepper, garlic, and artichoke hearts and let the whole thing simmer for 5 minutes or so.

Check on the bacon while the beef is simmering. If it's not crisp yet, give it another minute or so.

Divide the beef mixture between 6 serving plates or bowls and crumble about a strip and a half of bacon over each portion before serving.

Yield: 6 servings, each with 9 grams of carbohydrates and 4 grams of fiber, for a total of 5 grams of usable carbs and 23 grams of protein.

⊕ Tex-Mex Skillet Lasagna

This will take every second of the fifteen minutes, but it's worth it. Not only is it yummy as can be, it'll feed at least 6 people, and I'm betting even the carbivores will eat it with no complaints. Go for it. And keep in mind that keeping that tilted lid on the skillet every possible second is the key to getting it done fast.

> 1 pound (455 g) ground chuck
>
> 1 small onion
>
> 8 ounces (225 g) cream cheese, softened
>
> 1 cup (225 g) cottage cheese
>
> 1 1/2 cups (173 g) 4 cheese Mexican blend
>
> 1 teaspoon cumin
>
> 1 1/3 cups (327 g) no-sugar-added spaghetti sauce
>
> 2/3 cup (173 g) salsa
>
> 1 1/2 tablespoons (12 g) chili powder
>
> 1 can black soy beans (Eden cans these.)
>
> 2 packets tofu shirataki noodles, fettuccini style

Put the biggest skillet you can get your hands on over medium-high heat and throw in the ground chuck. Spread it over the whole bottom of the skillet, for maximum heat exposure, and cover with a tilted lid.

Throw the onion in your food processor and chop it to a medium-fine consistency. Dump it in with the ground beef and stir it all up, turning the beef and breaking it up. Re-cover with that tilted lid.

Mix together the cream cheese, cottage cheese, 1/2 cup (58 g) of the 4 cheese Mexican blend, and the cumin. Set aside.

Go stir up your beef and onion and re-cover with that tilted lid! Now measure the spaghetti sauce and salsa together in a 2 cup (475 ml) measuring cup and assuming most of the pink is gone from your beef—it should be—stir it in. Go ahead and stir in the chili powder, too. Re-cover with the tilted lid!

Open your soy beans and drain. Add them to the skillet and re-cover!

Drain your shirataki, rinse them quick, and snip across them 5 or 6 times with your kitchen shears. Go stir them into the mixture in the skillet, which will be getting mighty full—this completely filled my big cast iron skillet.

Spoon the cream/cottage cheese mixture over the top and then sprinkle the rest of the 4 cheese blend over the top. Re-cover with that tilted lid and let it finish out the cooking time or until the 4 cheese blend is melty and then serve.

Yield: At least 6 servings, assuming 6, each will have 420 calories, 31 grams fat, 24 grams protein, 13 grams carbohydrate, 4 grams dietary fiber, and 9 grams usable carb.

⏱ Kinda Cajun Skillet Supper

This is another recipe that takes multi-tasking, but it'll feed the family on a pound of ground chuck. This would also be good with pork sausage instead.

> 1 pound (455 g) ground chuck
>
> 1/2 head cauliflower
>
> 1 celery rib
>
> 1 medium onion
>
> 1 medium green pepper
>
> 2 teaspoons chopped garlic
>
> 5 bacon slices
>
> 1/2 cup (55 g) chopped roasted and salted pecans
>
> 5 teaspoons (15 g) Cajun seasoning
>
> 2 teaspoons beef bouillon granules
>
> Louisiana-style hot sauce

First put your biggest skillet over medium-high heat and start the ground beef browning; break it up to cover the whole bottom of the skillet. Cover with a tilted lid.

Whack the cauliflower into chunks and run it through the shredding blade of your food processor. Put the cauli-rice in a microwaveable casserole with a lid, add a couple of tablespoons (28 ml) water, cover, and nuke on high for 6 minutes.

Go stir your beef! Now swap out the shredding blade of your food processor for the S-blade. Whack the celery, onion, and pepper into hunks, throw them in, and pulse to chop to a medium consistency.

Check your beef. If you think there's too much grease, pour some off, but leave at least a few tablespoons (45 to 60 ml). Dump in the veggies and add the garlic, too. Stir it all together and put that tilted lid back on.

Lay the bacon slices on a microwave bacon rack or in a Pyrex pie plate; you want them ready to swap out with the cauliflower as soon as the microwave beeps! Then chop your pecans.

By now your cauliflower is done. Pull it out, stick the bacon in, and set the timer for 5 to 6 minutes. Drain your cauliflower and dump it in the skillet.

Add the Cajun seasoning and beef bouillon concentrate to the skillet and stir everything together really well until the seasonings are evenly distributed.

Stir in the pecans and dish it up.

When the bacon is done, use your kitchen shears to snip a slice over each serving and eat.

Yield: 4 to 5 servings, assuming 5, each will have 399 calories, 30 grams fat, 21 grams protein, 12 grams carbohydrate, 4 grams dietary fiber, and 8 grams usable carb.

⊕ Sweet and Sour Pork

This is not exactly authentic because the pork isn't battered and fried. Still, it tastes great! And it's far lower-carb than Sweet and Sour from a Chinese restaurant. If it feels strange to you not to serve this stir-fry over something, there's no reason not to make some cauliflower "rice" to serve with it.

3 tablespoons (45 ml) rice or cider vinegar

1 1/2 tablespoons (2.3 g) Splenda

3 tablespoons (45 g) canned, crushed pineapple in juice

1 teaspoon soy sauce

1/4 teaspoon blackstrap molasses

1/2 teaspoon minced garlic

3 tablespoons (45 ml) oil

12 ounces (340 g) boneless pork loin, cut into thin strips

1/2 medium green pepper, cut into squares

1/2 medium onion, sliced

Guar or xanthan

Mix together the vinegar, Splenda, pineapple, soy sauce, molasses, and garlic and set it by the stove.

Heat the oil in a wok or large skillet over highest heat. Add the pork and stir-fry until it's half-done. Add the peppers and onions and keep stir-frying. When all the pink is gone from the pork, add the vinegar mixture and stir. Let the whole thing simmer for a couple of minutes, stirring once or twice, until the vegetables are tender-crisp. Thicken the pan juices just a touch with guar or xanthan and serve.

Yield: 2 or 3 servings. Assuming 2 servings, each will have 11 grams of carbohydrates and 1 gram of fiber, for a total of 10 grams of usable carbs and 36 grams of protein.

✳ Each serving also packs 782 milligrams of potassium!

⊕ Sweet and Sour Chicken

No big surprise—you can make the same recipe with chicken, instead.

Make the recipe for *Sweet and Sour Pork*, substituting 12 ounces (340 g) of boneless, skinless chicken breast for the pork.

Yield: 2 or 3 servings. Assuming 2 servings, each will have 11 grams of carbohydrates and 1 gram of fiber, for a total of 10 grams of usable carbs and 39 grams of protein.

✻ The potassium content drops a bit, but you'll still get 479 milligrams.

⊕ Mediterranean Turkey Stir Fry

This dish is full of bright, glorious flavors!

1 1/2 pounds (680 g) boneless turkey tenderloin, sliced very thinly
3 to 4 tablespoons (45 to 60 ml) olive oil
1 medium onion, sliced
1 medium green pepper, cut into strips
1/4 cup (60 ml) dry white wine
1/4 cup (60 ml) lemon juice
1 can (2.25 ounces, or 70 g) sliced ripe olives, drained
2 teaspoons minced garlic or 4 cloves garlic, crushed
1 teaspoon dried oregano
2 teaspoons chicken bouillon concentrate
Guar or xanthan
4 tablespoons (16 g) fresh chopped parsley

In a large skillet or wok, start stir-frying the turkey in the olive oil over high heat. When it's about half-done (half the pink is gone), add the onion and pepper. Continue stir-frying until all the pink is gone from the turkey.

Add the wine, lemon juice, olives, garlic, oregano, and bouillon and let the whole thing cook, stirring now and then, for another 3 to 4 minutes or until the vegetables are tender-crisp. Thicken the pan juices slightly with the guar or xanthan. Turn off the burner, stir in the parsley, and serve.

Yield: 4 servings, each with 8 grams of carbohydrates and 2 grams of fiber, for a total of 6 grams of usable carbs and 39 grams of protein.

⊕ Chicken Asparagus Stir-Fry

1 pound (455 g) asparagus

1 medium onion

8 ounces (225 g) canned sliced water chestnuts, drained

¼ cup (60 ml) dry sherry

¼ cup (60 ml) soy sauce

1 teaspoon minced garlic or 2 cloves garlic, crushed

1 ½ pounds (680 g) boneless, skinless chicken breast, sliced into thin strips

¼ cup (60 ml) oil

Guar or xanthan

Snap the ends off the asparagus where they break naturally and slice diagonally into ½-inch (1.3 cm) lengths. Slice the onion into thin half-rounds. Open the water chestnuts and drain them. Mix together the sherry, soy sauce, and garlic and have it sitting by the stove.

Heat the oil in a wok or large skillet over highest heat. Add the chicken and stir-fry for 2 to 3 minutes or until about half the pink is gone. Add the asparagus and onion and continue stir-frying until the chicken is cooked through.

Add the water chestnuts and the sherry mixture, stir to combine, and let the whole thing simmer for another 2 to 4 minutes or until the asparagus is bright green and tender-crisp. Thicken the juices just a little with the guar or xanthan and serve.

Yield: 4 or 5 servings. Assuming 4 servings, each will have 15 grams of carbohydrates and 3 grams of fiber, for a total of 12 grams of usable carbs and 41 grams of protein.

⏲ Ham and Beans Skillet

This is very down-home, which is often a good thing. My husband loves it. You can double this if you like, but your beans will take longer to microwave, possibly taking you a minute or two past the 15-minute mark. Even doubled, though, it's a good, fast supper!

6 ounces (170 g) cooked ham, cut into 1/2-inch (1.3 cm) cubes

1 tablespoon (14 g) butter or (15 ml) oil

2 cups (248 g) frozen cross-cut green beans

1 tablespoon (15 g) canned, crushed pineapple in juice

1 tablespoon (16 g) low-carbohydrate barbecue sauce

1/4 teaspoon grated gingerroot

1/2 teaspoon spicy brown mustard

Start to sauté the ham in the butter or oil over medium heat—you're just browning it a little. While that's happening, put the beans in a microwaveable casserole, add a couple of tablespoons (28 ml) of water, cover, and microwave on High for 7 minutes.

When the microwave goes "ding," check that the beans are done; if they're not, stir them and give them another 2 to 3 minutes. When they're just tender, drain them and add them to the browned ham cubes in the skillet. Add the pineapple, barbecue sauce, gingerroot, and mustard and stir well. Let it cook for just a minute to blend the flavors and then serve.

Yield: 2 servings, each with 13 grams of carbohydrates and 4 grams of fiber, for a total of 9 grams of usable carbs and 19 grams of protein.

⏲ Ham-Cheddar-Spinach Skillet Supper

This includes just about everything my husband likes best. No wonder he gave it a 10!

10 ounces (280 g) frozen chopped spinach

1 tablespoon (14 g) butter

1/2 medium onion

1/2 pound (225 g) cooked ham, cut into 1/2-inch (1.3 cm) cubes

1 cup (58 g) shredded cheddar cheese

1/2 cup (120 ml) heavy cream

1 tablespoon (11 g) spicy brown mustard

3 hard-boiled eggs

Put your spinach in a microwaveable casserole with a lid, add a few tablespoons (45 to 60 ml) of water, and cover. Nuke on high according to package directions, probably 5 to 7 minutes.

Put your big, heavy skillet over medium heat and throw in the butter.

Chop your half an onion—you can use your food processor, but for just a half an onion I used a knife and a cutting board because I needed them to cube the ham anyway. Slosh the melting butter around in the skillet and throw in the onion.

Now cube your ham and throw it in the skillet, too. Stir it up with the onion.

If you didn't buy preshredded cheddar, shred some quick. Measure your cream, too.

Okay, microwave beeped; your spinach is done. Drain it well—press it to get out extra water—then dump it in the skillet. Stir the spinach up with the ham and onions. Now stir in the cheese and cream. Measure in the mustard and stir that in, too.

Bring the whole thing to a simmer, stirring occasionally, while you peel the eggs.

When the cheese is melted and the sauce is creamy, dish it up. Then slice a hard-boiled egg over each bowlful and serve. (You could grate or chop the eggs instead, if you find it easier; I just like the pretty circles of white and yellow on top.)

Yield: 3 servings, each with 572 calories, 45 grams fat, 33 grams protein, 10 grams carbohydrate, 3 grams dietary fiber, and 7 grams usable carb.

Note: This is a great way to use up leftover ham, but you can also buy a hunk of precooked ham and use that. It's handy stuff, that precooked ham.

⊕ Poultry Hash

This is only a 15-minute recipe if you have leftover turkey or chicken in the house, but you'll be glad to have it that Monday after Thanksgiving when you've gone back to work and come home to find still more turkey needing to be used up! This tastes good made with the remains of a rotisseried chicken, too.

> 1/4 head cauliflower
>
> 1 medium turnip (a little bigger than a tennis ball)
>
> 1/2 medium onion, diced
>
> 1 tablespoon (14 g) butter
>
> 2 cups (280 g) diced leftover turkey or chicken
>
> 3/4 cup (175 ml) half-and-half
>
> 1/2 teaspoon chicken bouillon concentrate
>
> 1/2 teaspoon poultry seasoning
>
> Guar or xanthan (optional)
>
> Salt and pepper

Whack the cauliflower into a few big chunks and drop it into a food processor with the S-blade in place. Peel the turnip, whack it into quarters, and throw it in there, too. Pulse until everything's chopped to a medium consistency. Dump it into a microwaveable casserole with a lid, add a couple of tablespoons (28 ml) of water, cover it, and nuke it on High for 7 minutes.

Meanwhile, in a big, heavy skillet, start sautéing the onion in the butter over medium heat. While that sautés, dice the leftover fowl.

Add the turkey or chicken to the skillet and stir it into the onion. By now the cauliflower and turnip should be done; pull them out of the microwave, drain them, and add them to the skillet, too. Stir in the half-and-half, bouillon, and poultry seasoning, cover it, and let it simmer for just a minute or two to make sure everything is hot all the way through. Thicken it just a tad, if you like, with the guar or xanthan, salt and pepper to taste, and serve.

Yield: 3 servings, each with 8 grams of carbohydrates and 1 gram of fiber, for a total of 7 grams of usable carbs and 24 grams of protein.

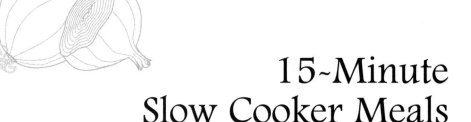

15-Minute Slow Cooker Meals

Okay, I admit it—none of the recipes in this chapter is done in 15 minutes. But that doesn't keep them from being just as convenient—or even more so!—than the recipes in the rest of the book, since they cook happily by themselves while you're out having a life.

With these recipes, the 15-minute limit is on preparation time, not cooking time. All of these recipes require no more than 15 minutes hands-on time, both before cooking and after cooking combined. No spending a half-hour dredging little bits of meat in flour and browning them before you can get your dinner in the slow cooker and your butt out the door, and no coming home from a long day's work to a houseful of hungry people, only to have to add things to your slow cooker meal and then wait an extra half hour. Nope, all these recipes truly are fast and simple—and tasty!

By the way, it's good to know how to speed up or slow down slow cooker food, should you need to: If you want to cut a good hour off your slow cooker recipe, put everything in the crockery liner, put the crockery liner in your microwave oven (this assumes, of course, that your crockery liner lifts out of the electric base, and fits in your microwave—mine does both), and microwave it on 50 percent power for 5 to 10 minutes—just long enough to warm everything through. Then put the crockery liner in the base, cover, and set as per the recipe. To slow a recipe down, you can put the meat in frozen! This will add a good 2 to 3 hours to your cooking time.

⊕ 3-Minute Slow Cooker Pot Roast

This recipe is very 1965, but it's still incredibly easy and it tastes great. Puréed cauliflower "fauxtatoes" are nice with this—they give you something to put the gravy on.

> 8 ounces (225 g) sliced mushrooms
> 2 to 3 pound (0.9 to 1.3 kg) boneless chuck pot roast
> 1 envelope French Onion soup mix
> 1/2 cup (120 ml) dry red wine
> Guar or xanthan

Dump the mushrooms in the bottom of your slow cooker and plunk the roast on top of them. Mix together the onion soup mix and wine and pour it over the whole thing. Slap on the lid, set the slow cooker to Low, and forget about it for 8 hours.

When you come home, fish out the roast (carefully—it will be very tender) and use the guar or xanthan to thicken up the juices in the slow cooker. Serve this gravy with the pot roast.

Yield: Assuming a 2-pound roast (900 g), this will yield 6 servings. If you eat every drop of the gravy, each serving will have 6 grams of carbohydrates and 1 gram of fiber, for a total of 5 grams of usable carbs and 25 grams of protein.

⊕ Pepperoncini Beef

Pepperoncini are hot-but-not-scorching pickled Italian salad peppers
—you'll find these in the same aisle as the olives and pickles—and they
make this beef very special.

> 2 to 3 pounds (0.9 to 1.3 kg) boneless chuck pot roast
>
> 1 cup (225 g) pepperoncini peppers, with the vinegar they're packed in
>
> 1/2 medium onion, chopped
>
> Guar or xanthan
>
> Salt and pepper

Slap the beef in the slow cooker, pour the pepperoncini on top, and strew the onion over that. Put on the lid, set the slow cooker to Low, and leave it for 8 hours.

When it's done, fish out the meat, put it on a platter, and use a slotted spoon to fish out the peppers and pile them on top of the roast. Thicken the juices in the pot with the guar or xanthan, salt and pepper to taste, and serve with the roast.

Yield: Assuming a 2-pound roast (900 g), this will yield 6 servings, each with 3 grams of carbohydrates, a trace of fiber, and 24 grams of protein.

☺ Caribbean Slow Cooker Lamb

I buy whole legs of lamb and have the butcher at the grocery store cut them up for me—a smallish roast from each end and steaks from the middle. They never charge for this service, and this gives me lamb roasts small enough to fit in my slow cooker. The problem ingredient here is the tamarind concentrate—look in a grocery store with a good International section. I found it in a medium-size town in southern Indiana, so you may well find it near you! If you can't find it, you could use a tablespoon (15 ml) of lemon juice and a teaspoon of Splenda instead, and your lamb will be less authentically Caribbean-tasting but still yummy.

2- to 3-pound (0.9 to 1.3 kg) section of a leg of lamb

1/2 medium onion, chopped

1/2 teaspoon minced garlic or 1 clove garlic, crushed

1 teaspoon tamarind concentrate

1 tablespoon (11 g) spicy brown mustard

1 cup (160 g) canned diced tomatoes

1 teaspoon hot sauce—preferably Caribbean Scotch Bonnet
  sauce—or more or less, to taste

Guar or xanthan

Salt and pepper

Place the lamb in the slow cooker. Stir together the onion, garlic, tamarind, mustard, tomatoes, and hot sauce and pour over the lamb. Set the cooker on Low and let it cook for a good 8 hours.

When it's done, remove the lamb to a serving platter, thicken the pot juices with the guar or xanthan if it seems necessary, salt and pepper to taste, and serve.

Yield: Assuming a 2 1/2-pound (1.1 kg) section of a leg of lamb, this will be 6 servings, each with 5 grams of carbohydrates and a trace of fiber (if you eat all the gravy—fewer carbs if you don't), and 27 grams of protein.

⊕ Slow Cooker Chicken Guadeloupe

This isn't authentically anything, but it borrows its flavors from the Creole cooking of the Caribbean.

> 1 cut-up broiler-fryer chicken, about 3 1/2 pounds (1.6 kg), or whatever chicken parts you prefer
>
> 1/2 medium onion, chopped
>
> 2 teaspoons ground allspice
>
> 1 teaspoon dried thyme
>
> 1/4 cup (60 ml) lemon juice; bottled is fine
>
> 1 can (14 ounces, or 400 g) diced tomatoes with chilies
>
> 1 shot (3 tablespoons, or 45 ml) dark rum
>
> Guar or xanthan
>
> Salt and pepper

Just throw the chicken, onion, allspice, thyme, lemon juice, chilies, and rum in the slow cooker, set it to Low, and let it go for 5 to 6 hours. Fish out the chicken carefully—it'll be sliding from the bone! Thicken up the stuff in the pot with the guar or xanthan, salt and pepper to taste, and serve over the chicken.

Yield: 5 or 6 servings. Assuming 5 servings, each will have 6 grams of carbohydrates and 1 gram of fiber, for a total of 5 grams of usable carbs and 35 grams of protein.

⊕ Sort of Ethiopian Chicken Stew

Again, the slow cooker method is hardly authentic, but the flavors come from an Ethiopian recipe—except that the Ethiopians would use a lot more cayenne! Increase it if you like really hot food.

> 1 cut-up broiler-fryer, about 3 pounds (1.3 kg)
>
> 1 medium onion, chopped
>
> 1 teaspoon cayenne
>
> 1 teaspoon paprika
>
> 1/2 teaspoon pepper
>
> 1/2 teaspoon grated gingerroot
>
> 2 tablespoons (28 ml) lemon juice
>
> 1/2 cup (120 ml) water
>
> Guar or xanthan
>
> Salt and pepper

Throw the chicken, onion, cayenne, paprika, pepper, gingerroot, lemon juice, and water in your slow cooker and set it to Low. Leave it for 5 to 6 hours. If you'd like to make this really stewlike, you can pick the meat off the bones when it's done (which will be very easy), thicken the gravy with guar or xanthan, and then stir the chicken back into the liquid. Or you can just serve the gravy over the chicken. Take your pick.

Yield: 5 or 6 servings. Assuming 5 servings, each will have 3 grams of carbohydrates and 1 gram of fiber, for a total of 2 grams of usable carbs and 35 grams of protein.

⏲ Chipotle Turkey Legs

This dish has spicy, rich Southwestern flavor.

 3 turkey legs

 1 1/2 teaspoons cumin

 1 teaspoon chili powder

 1 teaspoon dried, powdered sage

 1 teaspoon minced garlic or 2 cloves garlic, crushed

 1/2 teaspoon red pepper flakes

 1/4 teaspoon turmeric

 1 or 2 canned chipotle chilies in adobo sauce, plus a couple
   of teaspoons of the sauce they come in

 8 ounces (225 g) tomato sauce

 1 tablespoon (15 ml) Worcestershire sauce

 6 tablespoons (42 g) shredded queso quesadilla cheese (optional)*

 Guar or xanthan

* This is a mild, white Mexican cheese. Monterey Jack is an acceptable substitute.

Plunk the turkey legs in the slow cooker. (If you can fit more, feel free. My slow cooker will only hold 3.) Put the cumin, chili powder, sage, garlic, red pepper flakes, turmeric, chilies, tomato sauce, and Worcestershire sauce in the blender, run it for a minute, and then pour the mixture over the turkey legs. Cover, turn the slow cooker to Low, and leave it for 5 to 6 hours.

When it's done, remove each turkey leg to a serving plate, thicken the juices in the pot with guar or xanthan, and spoon over the turkey legs. If you like, sprinkle 2 tablespoons (14 g) of shredded cheese over each turkey leg and let it melt for a minute or two before serving.

Yield: 3 servings, each with 8 grams of carbohydrates and 2 grams of fiber, for a total of 6 grams of usable carbs and—depending on the size of the turkey legs—40 to 50 grams of protein.

Note: Chipotle peppers are smoked jalapeños. They're very different from regular jalapeños, and they're quite delicious. Look for them, canned in adobo sauce, in the Mexican foods section of big grocery stores. Since you're unlikely to use the whole can at once, you'll be happy to know that you can store your chipotles in the freezer, where they'll live happily for months and stay pliable enough that you can peel one off when you want to use it.

☺ Choucroute Garni

This is a streamlined version of a traditional dish from the Alsace region of France—the name means Garnished Sauerkraut. It's so simple and so good, especially on a cold night.

1 can (14 ounces, or 400 g) can red sauerkraut

1 tablespoon (15 g) bacon grease

1/4 cup (60 ml) apple cider vinegar

1 tablespoon (1.5 g) Splenda

1/2 medium onion, thinly sliced

2 tablespoons (28 ml) gin

1/4 cup (60 ml) dry white wine

1 pound (455 g) meat—your choice of any combination of kielbasa, smoked sausage, frankfurters, link sausages, 1/4-inch thick (6 mm) ham slices, or smoked pork chops*

* I use 1/2 pound (225 g) each of the lowest carbohydrate kielbasa and smoked sausage I can find.

Dump your sauerkraut into a colander, rinse lightly, drain, and dump into the slow cooker. Add the bacon grease, vinegar, Splenda, onion, gin, and wine and give it a quick stir. Plunk the meat on top, cover the slow cooker, and set it to Low. Cook for 5 to 6 hours.

Yield: 3 or 4 servings. Assuming 3 servings and depending on what meats you use, each will have in the neighborhood of 9 grams of carbohydrates and 3 grams of fiber, for a total of 6 grams of usable carbs (you can cut this by using the very lowest carbohydrate sausages you can find) and roughly 16 grams of protein.

Note: This doesn't even start to fill my slow cooker, so feel free to double or even triple this recipe. If you increase it, I'd layer it—a layer of kraut, a layer of meat, a layer of kraut, and so on. And, of course, you'll have to increase the cooking time by an hour, maybe two, depending on how many extra layers you use.

Slow Cooker Ribs

We just love ribs around here, but I've never thought of them as something "quick and easy." Then I thought of putting them in the slow cooker. Wow!

Slow cooker ribs aren't exactly like ribs done over a slow fire, of course, but they're incredibly tasty and falling-off-the-bone tender. What's more, they're really, really easy. Here are a few ideas on how to cook ribs in a slow cooker.

⊕ Rosemary-Ginger Ribs with Apricot Glaze

Blue Slaw—or any coleslaw—is good with these. Also, feel free to use a full-size slab of ribs—about 6 pounds (2.7 kg) worth—and double the seasonings if you're feeding a family.

> 1 slab baby back ribs, about 2 1/2 pounds (1.1 kg)
>
> Purchased Rosemary-Ginger Rub (Stubb's makes this)
>
> 2 tablespoons (40 g) low-sugar apricot preserves
>
> 1 1/2 teaspoons spicy brown mustard
>
> 1 teaspoon Splenda
>
> 1 1/2 teaspoons soy sauce

Sprinkle both sides of the slab of ribs generously with the Rosemary-Ginger Rub. Curl the slab of ribs around and fit it down into your slow cooker. Cover and set the slow cooker on Low. Forget about it for 9 to 10 hours. (No, I didn't forget anything. You don't put any liquid in the slow cooker. Don't sweat it.)

When the time's up, mix together the preserves, mustard, Splenda, and soy sauce. Carefully remove the ribs from the slow cooker—they may fall apart on you a bit, they'll be so tender. Arrange them meaty-side-up on a broiler rack. Spread the apricot glaze evenly over the ribs and run them under a broiler set on High, 3 to 4 inches (7.5 to 10 cm) from the heat, for 7 to 8 minutes, and then serve.

Yield: 2 or 3 servings. Assuming 3 servings, each will have 5 grams of carbohydrates, a trace of fiber, and 38 grams of protein.

⊕ Slow Cooker "Barbecued" Ribs

Okay, it's not really barbecue because it's not done over a fire. But this recipe tastes great and lets you dig into your ribs within minutes of walking in the door.

>   1 slab baby back ribs, about 2 1/2 pounds (1.1 kg)
>
>   *Memphis-Style Dry Rub* (page 306, or you can purchase good
>   dry rub in most grocery stores)
>
>   1/4 cup (65 g) *Reduced-Carb Spicy Barbecue Sauce* (see page 311)
>   or 1/4 cup (65 g) purchased low-carb barbecue sauce*

* Atkins makes one, and so does Walden—these are both available through online retailers. There's also a brand called Stubb's, pretty widely distributed in grocery stores, that has less than half the sugar of most commercial barbecue sauces and tastes great. That's what I use.

Sprinkle the slab of ribs liberally on both sides with the dry rub, coil the ribs up, and slide them into your slow cooker. Cover, set to Low, and let them go for 9 to 10 hours.

When dinnertime rolls around, pull the ribs out of the slow cooker—as in the previous recipe, do this carefully because they'll be falling-apart tender. Lay the ribs on a broiler rack, meaty side up, and spread the barbecue sauce over them. Broil 3 to 4 inches (7.5 to 10 cm) from the broiler set on High for 7 to 8 minutes, and then serve.

Yield: Your carb count will be a bit different depending on whether you use homemade sugar-free barbecue sauce or commercial low-carb sauce. If 3 people share these, each will get about 5 grams of carbohydrates, no fiber, and 38 grams of protein.

Note: If you'd like to give these a smoked flavor, you can buy liquid smoke flavoring at your grocery store. Simply brush the ribs with the liquid smoke before you sprinkle on the dry rub.

◷ Slow Cooker Teriyaki Ribs

These are sweet, spicy and tangy and falling-off-the-bone tender. The 15-minute time frame does not include making the ketchup, but the teriyaki sauce should fit in, and you'll want to have ketchup on hand all the time, anyway.

> 6 pounds (2.7 kg) pork spare ribs, cut into 3 or 4 pieces so they fit in the pot
> 3/4 cup (180 g) Dana's No-Sugar Ketchup or commercial no-sugar ketchup
> 1 batch *Teriyaki Sauce* (see page 313)
> 1/4 cup (6 g) Splenda
> 1/4 teaspoon blackstrap molasses
> 1 teaspoon minced garlic or 2 cloves garlic, crushed
> Guar or xanthan

Plop the ribs in the slow cooker. Mix the ketchup, teriyaki sauce, Splenda, molasses, and garlic together, pour it into the cooker, cover the pot, and set it on Low. Forget it for 10 hours.

When the time's up, use tongs to pull out the now unbelievably tender and flavorful ribs. Ladle out as much of the pot liquid as you think you'll use and thicken it using the guar or xanthan. Serve the sauce over the ribs.

Yield: 6 servings, each with roughly 3 grams of carbohydrates, a trace of fiber (depending on how much of the liquid you eat), and 48 grams of protein.

☺ "I've Got a Life" Chicken

This is remarkably good—sweet and tangy and fruity. It takes just about the whole 15 minutes—about 12 to get it into the pot and another couple at the far end for thickening the sauce—but it's worth it.

> 3 to 3 1/2 pounds (1.3 to 1.6 kg) bone-in chicken parts of your choice—I use legs
>   and thighs, but a whole cut up chicken would work great.
>
> 8 ounces (225 g) sliced mushrooms
>
> 3 tablespoons (45 ml) orange juice
>
> Grated zest of one orange
>
> 1 tablespoon (6 g) chicken bouillon concentrate
>
> 1/2 teaspoon pepper
>
> 1 can (8 ounces, or 225 g) can tomato sauce
>
> 2 tablespoons (28 ml) soy sauce
>
> 2 tablespoons (3 g) Splenda
>
> 1/2 teaspoon blackstrap molasses
>
> 2 teaspoons minced garlic or 4 cloves garlic, crushed
>
> 1 teaspoon dried thyme
>
> Guar or xanthan

Remove the skin and any big lumps of fat from the chicken and throw it in the slow cooker. (You can save time by buying chicken with the skin already removed, but it's more expensive.) Dump the mushrooms on top.

Mix together the orange juice, orange zest, bouillon, pepper, tomato sauce, soy sauce, Splenda, molasses, garlic, and thyme and dump it on top of the chicken and mushrooms. Cover the pot, set it to Low, and let it cook for 5 to 6 hours.

When it's done, pull the chicken out and put it on a platter. Use the guar or xanthan to thicken up the sauce in the pot and serve it with the chicken.

Yield: 5 or 6 servings. Assuming 6 servings, each will have 8 grams of carbohydrates and 1 gram of fiber, for a total of 7 grams of usable carbs (assuming you eat all of the gravy) and 31 grams of protein.

☺ Slow Cooker Brewery Chicken and Vegetables

There are plenty of vegetables in here, so you don't need a thing with it, except maybe some bread for the carb-eaters in the family. And the gravy comes out a beautiful color!

8 ounces (225 g) turnips (two turnips roughly the size of tennis balls), peeled and cut in chunks

2 stalks celery, sliced

1 medium carrot, scrubbed and sliced

1/2 medium onion, sliced

1 tablespoon (6 g) chicken bouillon concentrate

2 1/2 to 3 pounds (1.1 to 1.3 kg) cut-up chicken—I use leg and thigh quarters, cut apart at the joint.

1 can (12 ounces, or 355 ml) very low-carb light beer—Miller Lite, Milwaukee's Best Light, or Michelob Ultra

1 can (14.5 ounces, or 410 g) can diced tomatoes with green chilies

Guar or xanthan (optional)

Salt and pepper

Just put the turnips, celery, carrot, onion, bouillon, and chicken in the slow cooker in the order given. Pour the beer and the tomatoes over the lot, cover it, and set the slow cooker to Low. Cook for 8 to 9 hours.

When it's done, use tongs to pull out the chicken and place it on a serving platter. Then, using a slotted spoon, scoop out the vegetables. Put 1 1/2 cups (340 g) of them in the blender and pile the rest on and around the chicken on the platter. Scoop out 1 1/2 to 2 cups (355 to 475 ml) of the liquid left in the slow cooker and put it in the blender with the vegetables. Purée the veggies and broth and thicken the mixture a little more with the guar or xanthan, if it seems necessary. Salt and pepper to taste and serve as a sauce with the chicken and vegetables.

Yield: 5 or 6 servings. Assuming 5 servings, each will have 8 grams of carbohydrates and 2 grams of fiber, for a total of 6 grams of usable carbs and 36 grams of protein.

☉ Chicken Chili Verde

This is marvelous and a really nice change from the traditional beef chili.

1 1/2 pounds (680 g) boneless, skinless chicken breasts

1 1/2 cups (384 g) bottled salsa verde

1/2 medium onion, chopped

1 bay leaf

1/2 teaspoon pepper

1 teaspoon ground cumin

1 teaspoon minced garlic or 2 cloves garlic, crushed

1 to 2 tablespoons (9 to 18 g) jarred, sliced jalapeños*

2 teaspoons chicken bouillon concentrate

Guar or xanthan (optional)

Sour cream

Shredded Monterey Jack cheese

Chopped fresh cilantro

* I used 2 tablespoons (18 g), and it came out fairly hot.

Just plunk the chicken breasts into your slow cooker and throw the salsa verde, onion, bay leaf, pepper, cumin, garlic, jalapeños, and bouillon on top. Cover it, set it to Low, and let it cook for 9 to 10 hours.

When the time's up, take a fork and shred the chicken right there in the pot, which will now be very easy to do. Stir it up, thicken the chili a little with the guar or xanthan if you think it needs it, and serve with sour cream, shredded cheese, and chopped cilantro on top.

Yield: 5 servings, each with 7 grams of carbohydrates, a trace of fiber, and 31 grams of protein (before adding garnishes).

Note: Leftover Chicken Chili Verde makes great omelets, especially combined with Monterey Jack cheese!

15~Minute Side Dishes

I think these side dishes make very nice accompaniments to simple protein dishes—a grilled or pan-broiled steak or chop, a rotisserie chicken from the grocery store, or something like that. Of course, if you do both a 15-minute side dish *and* a 15-minute main course, you're looking at a bit more than 15 minutes total cooking time (although not necessarily 30 minutes, since you may well be able to multi-task).

When you *don't* feel like taking the time and effort to make one of these side dishes, or when your entire 15 minutes is going into making your main course, the easiest sides are frozen vegetables or bagged salad with bottled dressing. There is nothing wrong with either of these, and we'll talk a little about them at the end of the chapter.

We start this section with a couple of basic recipes that every low-carber needs. These are taken from my previous book, *500 Low-Carb Recipes*: *Fauxtatoes*, a cauliflower purée that makes a great substitute for mashed potatoes, and *Cauliflower "Rice,"* cauliflower run through the shredding blade of a food processor. These two recipes are repeated because they're great for serving with any dish that has a sauce or gravy. Either one of these is the obvious side, for instance, with any of the slow cooker dishes that makes a lot of good, flavorful gravy.

After these two recipes, you'll find a variety of ways to season *Cauliflower "Rice"*—I've become quite enchanted with this wonderful food, as you'll see! All these recipes start the same way—you run a half a head of cauliflower through a food processor's shredding blade and microwave it. If, like me, you discover that you're very fond of this wonderfully versatile food, you might consider running a couple of heads of cauliflower through the food processor over the weekend and storing the resultant cauliflower "rice" in a large zip-per-lock bag in the refrigerator to draw on through the week. However, all of these recipes fit into the 15-minute limit, including the minute or two needed to shred the cauliflower.

There are also recipes here where the cauliflower is sliced or chunked. Indeed, there are more recipes for cauliflower than any other vegetable here because cauliflower is The Great Fooler and makes a terrific substitute for rice, potatoes, and even bulgar wheat or noodles. And of course, cauliflower is more nutritious than any of these!

By the way, don't bother cutting the core out of the cauliflower—just trim off the leaves and the very base of the stem, whack the whole thing into chunks, and shred up the core and stem along with the flowerets. If you core the cauliflower, it will still work fine, but the yield for these recipes will be somewhat less.

⊕ Cauliflower Puree, a.k.a. Fauxtatoes

This is a wonderful substitute for mashed potatoes with any dish that has a gravy or sauce. Feel free, by the way, to use frozen cauliflower instead; it works quite well here.

> 1 head cauliflower or 1 1/2 pounds (680 g) frozen cauliflower
>
> 4 tablespoons (55 g) butter
>
> Salt and pepper

Put the cauliflower in a microwaveable casserole with a lid, add a couple of tablespoons (28 ml) of water, and cover. Nuke it on High for 10 to 12 minutes or until quite tender but not sulfury smelling. (You may steam or boil the cauliflower, if you prefer.) Drain it thoroughly and put it through the blender or food processor until it's well puréed. Add butter, salt, and pepper to taste.

Yield: At least 6 generous servings, each with 5 grams of carbohydrates and 2 grams of fiber, for a total of 3 grams of usable carbs and 2 grams of protein.

☉ Fauxtatoes with Chèvre and Peas

This is an unexpected upgrade to *Fauxtatoes*, and the textural and color contrast of the peas adds a lot of interest.

> ¹/₂ head cauliflower
> ¹/₂ cup (75 g) frozen peas
> 4 ounces (115 g) chèvre (goat) cheese
> salt and pepper

Microwave cauliflower as for *Fauxtatoes*. See page 232.

In the meantime, put the peas in a small, microwaveable dish, add a teaspoon or so of water, and cover.

When the cauliflower comes out of the microwave, put the peas in and give them just 2 minutes on high.

In the meantime, drain and puree the cauliflower with the chèvre. When the peas are done, stir them in, too (don't puree!), salt and pepper to taste, and serve.

Yield: 4 servings, each with 108 calories, 6 grams fat, 8 grams protein, 6 grams carbohydrate, 3 grams dietary fiber, and 3 grams usable carb.

☉ Cauliflower "Rice"

This is with thanks to Fran McCullough! I got this idea from her book *Living Low Carb*, and it's served me very well, indeed.

> ¹/₂ head cauliflower
> Butter (optional)

Simply put the cauliflower through your food processor using the shredding blade. This gives a texture that is remarkably similar to rice. You can steam this, microwave it, or even sauté it in butter. I virtually always microwave it, usually for 7 minutes on High, as you'll see in all the following recipes. Whatever you do, though, don't overcook it!

Yield: This is at least 3 or 4 servings. Assuming 3 servings, each will have 5 grams of carbohydrates and 2 grams of fiber, for a total of 3 grams of usable carbs and 2 grams of protein.

☉Blue Cheese-Scallion "Risotto"

Since West Coasters call scallions "green onions," I toyed with calling this "Blue-Green 'Risotto'." Making risotto out of cauliflower "rice" is one of the best ideas I've ever had!

> 1/2 head cauliflower
>
> 8 scallions, thinly sliced
>
> 2/3 cup (100 g) diced green bell pepper
>
> 1 tablespoon (14 g) butter
>
> 1 tablespoon (15 ml) olive oil
>
> 1 teaspoon chicken bouillon concentrate
>
> 1/4 cup (60 ml) dry white wine
>
> 1/4 cup (30 g) crumbled blue cheese
>
> 1/4 cup (25 g) grated Parmesan cheese
>
> 2 tablespoons (28 ml) heavy cream

Put the cauliflower through the food processor using the shredding blade. Put it in a microwaveable casserole, add a couple of tablespoons (28 ml) of water, cover, and microwave on High for 7 minutes.

While that's nuking, slice the scallions and dice the pepper. Then, in a large, heavy skillet over medium heat, start sautéing the scallions and pepper in the butter and oil.

When the microwave goes "ding," remove the cauliflower and drain it. When the green pepper is starting to get soft, add the cauliflower to the skillet and stir it in. Then stir in the bouillon, white wine, blue cheese, Parmesan cheese, and heavy cream. Cook for another 3 to 4 minutes and serve.

Yield: 5 servings, each with 4 grams of carbohydrates and 1 gram of fiber, for a total of 3 grams of usable carbs and 4 grams of protein.

⊕ Mushroom "Risotto"

Man, is this good! It's one of the best side dishes I've ever come up with.

1/2 head cauliflower

3 tablespoons (42 g) butter

1 cup (70 g) sliced mushrooms

1/2 medium onion, diced

1 teaspoon minced garlic or 2 cloves garlic

2 tablespoons (28 ml) dry vermouth

1 tablespoon (6 g) chicken bouillon concentrate

3/4 cup (75 g) grated Parmesan cheese

Guar or xanthan

2 tablespoons (8 g) chopped fresh parsley

Run the cauliflower through the food processor using the shredding blade. Put the cauliflower in a microwaveable casserole, add a couple of tablespoons (28 ml) of water, cover, and microwave on High for 7 minutes.

While the cauliflower is nuking, melt the butter over medium-high heat and add the mushrooms, onion, and garlic and sauté them all together.

When the cauliflower is done, pull it out of the microwave and drain it. When the mushrooms have changed color and are looking done, add the cauliflower and stir everything together. Stir in the vermouth, bouillon, and cheese and let the whole thing cook for another 2 to 3 minutes. Sprinkle just a little guar or xanthan over the "risotto," stirring all the while, to give it a creamy texture. Stir in the parsley and serve.

Yield: 5 servings, each with 4 grams of carbohydrates and 1 gram of fiber, for a total of 3 grams of usable carbs and 6 grams of protein.

☺ Artichoke "Risotto"

Bring home a rotisserie chicken from the grocery store, serve this along side it, and the family may get confused and think it's Sunday.

> 1/2 onion, diced
>
> 3 tablespoons (45 ml) olive oil
>
> 1/2 head cauliflower
>
> 1 cup (235 ml) dry white wine
>
> 3 teaspoons (6 g) chicken bouillon concentrate
>
> 1/2 teaspoon chopped garlic
>
> 2/3 cup (200 g) canned artichoke hearts, drained and chopped
>
> 1/2 cup (50 g) grated Parmesan cheese
>
> 2 tablespoons (28 ml) heavy cream
>
> salt and pepper to taste

First start the onion sautéing in the olive oil in a big, heavy saucepan over medium-low heat.

Trim the leaves and the very bottom of the stem off your half of a cauliflower and run it through the shredding blade of your food processor. Go stir your onions! You don't want them to brown.

Now dump the resulting cauli-rice into a microwaveable casserole with a lid (or you can place a microwaveable plate on top). Add a couple of tablespoons (28 ml) of water, cover, and nuke it for 6 minutes on high.

Okay, back to your sautéing onions. By now they should be turning translucent. Add the white wine, the bouillon concentrate, and the garlic and turn the burner up to high. You want to bring it to a boil and then turn the burner down just enough to keep the mixture boiling without boiling over.

While the wine mixture is reducing, chop your artichoke hearts and measure your Parmesan and cream.

Somewhere in here, your microwave will beep. Remove your cauli-rice and uncover it to stop the cooking.

When your wine has cooked down to about 1/4 of its original volume, add the cauli-rice, artichoke hearts, Parmesan, and cream. Stir it all up, salt and pepper to taste, and serve.

Yield: 5 servings, each with 195 calories, 13 grams fat, 6 grams protein, 7 grams carbohydrate, 2 grams dietary fiber, and 5 grams usable carb.

⊕ Saffron "Rice"

What a brilliant color this has! It looks so beautiful on your plate and is good with any main dish that's a little fruity-spicy.

1/2 head cauliflower

1 teaspoon saffron threads

1/4 cup (60 ml) water

1/2 medium onion, chopped

1 teaspoon minced garlic or 2 cloves garlic, crushed

2 tablespoons (28 g) butter

2 teaspoons chicken bouillon concentrate

1/4 cup (25 g) chopped toasted almonds

Run the cauliflower through the food processor using the shredding blade. Put the cauliflower in a microwaveable casserole, add a couple of tablespoons (28 ml) of water, cover, and microwave on High for 7 minutes.

Start soaking the saffron threads in the water. While that's happening, sauté the onion and garlic in the butter over medium heat in a large, heavy skillet.

When the cauliflower is done, remove it from the microwave, drain it, and add it to the skillet. Pour in the water and saffron and stir in the chicken bouillon concentrate. Let the whole thing cook together for a minute or two while you chop the almonds. Stir the almonds into the "rice" and serve.

Yield: 5 servings of brilliantly yellow "rice," each with 4 grams of carbohydrates and 1 gram of fiber, for a total of 3 grams of usable carbs and 2 grams of protein.

Variation: Traditionally, saffron rice has raisins in it. If you can afford the extra carbohydrates—if, for instance, you're serving a very low-carb main dish—you can stir in 3 tablespoons (27 g) of raisins with the saffron and water. Each serving of this version will have 8 grams of carbohydrates and 1 gram of fiber, for a total of 7 grams of usable carbs and 2 grams of protein.

Note: Saffron is the most expensive spice in the world and with good reason. Each saffron thread is the stamen of a particular kind of crocus flower. There are four per flower, and they all have to be plucked by hand with tweezers. It takes 50,000 of them to make a pound (455 g) of saffron! Luckily, small quantities of saffron make a big impact on a dish. Do look for saffron in a store that sells bulk spices—many health food stores do. At least that way you're not paying extra for that little glass jar.

⊕ Chicken-Almond "Rice"

This is great for all of you who miss Rice-a-Roni and similar products. And it's terrific with a simple rotisseried chicken.

> 1/2 head cauliflower
>
> 1/2 medium onion, chopped
>
> 2 tablespoons (28 g) butter
>
> 1 tablespoon (6 g) chicken bouillon concentrate
>
> 1 teaspoon poultry seasoning
>
> 1/4 cup (60 ml) dry white wine
>
> 1/4 cup (23 g) sliced or (28 g) slivered almonds

Run the cauliflower through the food processor using the shredding blade. Put the cauliflower in a microwaveable casserole, add a couple of tablespoons (28 ml) of water, cover, and microwave on High for 7 minutes.

While that's cooking, sauté the onion in 1 tablespoon (14 g) of butter in a large, heavy
skillet over medium-high heat.

When the cauliflower is done, pull it out of the microwave, drain it, and add it to the skillet. Add the chicken bouillon concentrate, poultry seasoning, and wine and stir. Turn the burner down to low heat.

Let that simmer for a minute or two while you sauté the almonds in the remaining tablespoon (14 g) of butter in a small, heavy skillet. When the almonds are golden, stir them into the "rice" and serve.

Yield: 5 servings, each with 4 grams of carbohydrates and 1 gram of fiber, for a total of 3 grams of usable carbs and 2 grams of protein.

Note: Sunkist now puts out sliced, toasted almonds in various flavors under the name "Almond Accents." Feel free to use these to vary this dish!

⊕ Beef and Bacon "Rice" with Pine Nuts

1/2 head cauliflower

4 strips bacon

1/2 medium onion, chopped

1 tablespoon (15 ml) beef bouillon concentrate

2 tablespoons (31 g) tomato sauce

2 tablespoons (18 g) toasted pine nuts

2 tablespoons (8 g) chopped fresh parsley

Run the cauliflower through the food processor using the shredding blade, put it in a microwaveable casserole, add a couple of tablespoons (28 ml) of water, cover it, and nuke it on High for 7 minutes.

While that's cooking, cut the bacon into little pieces—kitchen shears are good for this—and start the little bacon bits frying in a heavy skillet over medium-high heat. When a little grease has cooked out of the bacon, throw the onion into the skillet. Fry them until the onion is translucent and the bacon is browned and getting crisp.

By now the cauliflower should be done. Drain it and throw it in the skillet with the bacon and onion. Add the beef bouillon concentrate and tomato sauce and stir the whole thing up to combine everything—you can add a couple of tablespoons (28 ml) of water, if you like, to help the liquid flavorings spread.

Stir in the pine nuts and parsley (you can just snip it right into the skillet with those kitchen shears) and serve.

Yield: 4 or 5 servings. Assuming 4 servings, each will have 3 grams of carbohydrates and 1 gram of fiber, for a total of 2 grams of usable carbs and 4 grams of protein.

⏱ Alfredo in a Flash

This is so easy and so good! I figure this for two servings as a side dish, but with this carb and calorie count you could eat the whole thing. I like this for a hot snack.

> 1 package tofu shirataki, fettuccini width
>
> 1/4 cup (50 g) chive flavor whipped cream cheese
>
> 1 tablespoon (5 g) grated Parmesan cheese

Snip open your shirataki and dump them in a strainer. Give them a rinse, snip across them a couple of times with your kitchen shears, and plunk them in a microwave-able bowl. Nuke on high for a minute.

Pull your noodles out of the microwave and drain them again. Nuke a second time for a minute on high and drain again.

Stir in the chive cream cheese; it should melt into the hot noodles, but if you need to you could give the whole thing another 30 seconds in the microwave.

Stir in the Parmesan and serve.

Yield: 2 servings, each with 81 calories, 8 grams fat, 2 grams protein, 1 gram carbohydrate, trace dietary fiber, and 1 gram usable carb.

⊕ Sesame Noodles

Have you got a Chinese food jones? Here's your dish! This serves four as a side dish, but it makes a nice, light supper for two. And there's no law against halving the recipe if it's just you—but if you make the whole thing, you'll have leftovers to reheat tomorrow, you know.

    2 packages shirataki noodles, spaghetti width

    2 teaspoons chopped garlic

    2 tablespoons (28 ml) coconut oil

    2 tablespoons (32 g) natural peanut butter

    4 tablespoons (60 ml) rice vinegar

    4 tablespoons (60 ml) soy sauce

    2 tablespoons (28 ml) dark sesame oil

    2 tablespoons (3 g) Splenda, or the equivalent in liquid Splenda

    1/2 teaspoon chili garlic paste, or to taste

Drain and rinse the shirataki. Snip across them a few times, put them in a micro-waveable bowl big enough to eventually toss them in, and nuke them for 1 minute 30 seconds.

In the meantime, combine everything from the garlic through the chili paste in a small saucepan over low heat.

When the microwave beeps, re-drain the noodles, put them back in the bowl, and give them another 1 minute 30 seconds on high.

Whisk your sauce over low heat until it's smooth and thick—it won't take long.

When the microwave beeps again, drain the noodles one last time and put them back in their bowl. Pour on the sauce and toss.

Slice up the scallions really quick. Serve the noodles with the scallion scattered on top.

Yield: 4 servings, each with 205 calories, 18 grams fat, 4 grams protein, 9 grams carbohydrate, 3 grams dietary fiber, and 6 grams usable carb.

☉ Not-Quite-Middle-Eastern Salad

Here shredded cauliflower stands in for bulgar wheat instead of rice. This salad is incredibly delicious, incredibly nutritious, and quite beautiful on the plate. Plus it gets better after a couple of days in the fridge, so taking an extra few minutes to double the batch is definitely worth it.

> 1/2 head cauliflower
>
> 2/3 cup (93 g) sliced stuffed olives*
>
> 7 scallions, sliced
>
> 2 cups (60 g) triple-washed fresh spinach, finely chopped
>
> 1 stalk celery, diced
>
> 1 small ripe tomato, finely diced
>
> 4 tablespoons (16 g) chopped parsley
>
> 1/4 cup (60 ml) olive oil
>
> 1 teaspoon minced garlic or 2 cloves garlic, crushed
>
> 1 tablespoon (15 ml) red wine vinegar
>
> 2 tablespoons (28 g) mayonnaise
>
> Salt and pepper

*You can buy sliced stuffed olives in jars.

Run the cauliflower through the food processor using the shredding blade, put it in a microwaveable casserole, add a couple of tablespoons (28 ml) of water, cover the dish, and nuke it on High for just 5 minutes.

While that's cooking, put the olives, scallions, spinach, celery, tomato, and parsley in a large salad bowl.

When the cauliflower comes out of the microwave, dump it in a strainer and run cold water over it for a moment or two to cool it. (If you don't care about your salad being ready to eat in 15 minutes' time, you can let the cauliflower cool, uncovered, instead.) Drain the cauliflower well and dump it in with all the other vegetables. Add the oil, garlic, vinegar, and mayonnaise and toss. Salt and pepper to taste, toss again, and serve.

Yield: 6 servings, each with 5 grams of carbohydrates and 2 grams of fiber, for a total of 3 grams of usable carbs and 1 gram of protein.

⊕ Cauliflower Parmesan

This is wonderful with a simple broiled or grilled steak and easy to make while that steak is cooking.

 1/2 head cauliflower

 1/2 cup (120 ml) heavy cream

 1/2 cup (50 g) grated Parmesan cheese

 Salt and pepper

Run the cauliflower through the slicing disk on your food processor. Put it in a microwaveble casserole, add a couple of tablespoons (28 ml) of water, cover, and microwave on High for 4 minutes. When the cauliflower comes out of the micro-wave, drain it and put it in a large, heavy skillet you've sprayed with nonstick cook-ing spray. Reduce the heat to low. Add the cream and Parmesan, stir, cover, and let the whole thing simmer for 5 minutes or so. Salt and pepper to taste and then serve.

Yield: 4 servings, each with 2 grams of carbohydrates, a trace of fiber, and 5 grams of protein.

☉ Cauliflower Provencal

I had something similar to this at the Brattleboro, Vermont food coop and knew I could clone it. It's great hot or cold.

1/2 head cauliflower

24 cherry tomatoes

12 kalamata olives

1/4 cup (15 g) minced fresh parsley

2 tablespoons (18 g) capers, drained

6 tablespoons (90 ml) extra virgin olive oil

3 tablespoons (45 ml) lemon juice

1 teaspoon chopped garlic

salt and pepper

Whack your cauliflower into chunks about 1 to 2 inches (2.5 to 5 cm) across. Throw them in a microwaveable casserole with a lid, add a couple of tablespoons (28 ml) of water, cover, and nuke on high for ten minutes.

In the meantime, halve the cherry tomatoes, pit and chop the olives (just crush them with your thumb and flick out the pits), and chop the parsley. Throw it all in a big mixing bowl. Add the capers, too.

Measure and combine the olive oil, lemon juice, and garlic and mix together.

Okay, the cauliflower's done. Drain it well, add it to the bowl, and pour in the dressing. Toss it all up and serve hot or cold.

Yield: 4 to 5 servings, assuming 4, each will have 254 calories, 24 grams fat, 2 grams protein, 11 grams carbohydrate, 3 grams dietary fiber, and 8 grams usable carb.

☺Little Mama's Side Dish

This is just the thing with a simple dinner of broiled chops or a steak, and it's even good all by itself. It's beautiful to look at, too, what with all those colors.

4 slices bacon

1/2 head cauliflower

1/2 green pepper

1/2 medium onion

1/4 cup (35 g) sliced stuffed olives*

*You can buy sliced stuffed olives in jars.

Chop the bacon into small bits and start it frying in a large, heavy skillet over medium-high heat. (Give the skillet a squirt of nonstick cooking spray first.)

Chop the cauliflower into bits about 1/2 inch (1.3 cm) chunks. Chop up the stem, too; no need to waste it. Put the chopped cauliflower in a microwaveable casserole with a lid, add a couple of tablespoons (28 ml) of water, cover, and micro-wave for 7 minutes on High.

Give the bacon a stir; then it's back to the chopping board. Dice the pepper and onion. By now some fat has cooked out of the bacon and it is starting to brown around the edges. Add the pepper and onion to the skillet. Sauté until the onion is translucent and the pepper is starting to get soft.

By the time that confluence of events transpires, the cauliflower should be done. Add it to the skillet without draining, and stir—the extra little bit of water is going to help to dissolve the yummy bacon flavor from the bottom of the skillet and carry it through the dish.

Stir in the olives, let the whole thing cook another minute while stirring, and then serve.

Yield: 4 or 5 servings. Assuming 5 servings, each will have 3 grams of carbohydrates and 1 gram of fiber, for a total of 2 grams of usable carbs and 2 grams of protein.

☉ Easy Garlic Creamed Spinach

This is about the easiest creamed spinach ever and quite good too.

> 2 boxes (10 ounces, or 280 g) frozen chopped spinach, thawed
>   or 2 boxes (10 ounces, or 280 g) triple-washed fresh spinach
> 1 tablespoon (14 g) butter
> 1 package (5.2 ounces, or 145 g) creamy garlic-herb cheese, like
>   Boursin or Alouette

If you're using fresh spinach, you might coarsely chop it, quickly. Melt the butter in a large, heavy skillet and add the spinach. Cook, stirring, for 3 to 4 minutes—you want fresh spinach just barely wilted and frozen spinach just well-heated through.

Cut the cheese into a few chunks and add it to the skillet. Stir until the cheese is completely melted and then serve.

Yield: 6 servings, each with 4 grams of carbohydrates and 3 grams of fiber, for a total of 1 gram of usable carbs and 4 grams of protein.

⊕ Sour Cream Spinach

My husband liked this so much that he yummed down the whole batch.

> 1 package (10 ounces, or 280 g) package frozen chopped spinach
>
> 1/4 medium onion
>
> 2 tablespoons (28 g) butter
>
> 1/3 cup (77 g) sour cream
>
> 1 teaspoon cider vinegar

Unwrap the spinach and put it in a microwaveable casserole with a lid. Add a couple of tablespoons (28 ml) of water, cover, and zap it on High for 5 minutes.

Meanwhile, in a large, heavy skillet, start sautéing the onion in the butter over medium-high heat.

When the microwave goes "ding," check to see if the spinach is done—you want it good and hot right through but not cooked to death. If there's still a cold spot in the middle, stir it and put it back for another 2 minutes on High.

When the spinach is cooked and the onion is translucent, drain the spinach and stir it into the onion, combining well. Stir in the sour cream and the vinegar, heat it through without letting it simmer, and then serve.

Yield: 3 servings, each with 6 grams of carbohydrates and 3 grams of fiber, for a total of 3 grams of usable carbs and 4 grams of protein.

⊕ Spinach with Feta and Pine Nuts

This is good with any Mediterranean-style main dish.

10 ounces (280 g) frozen chopped spinach

1/2 medium onion

2 tablespoons (28 ml) olive oil

2 tablespoons (18 g) pine nuts, toasted (My grocery store carries them already toasted.)

1 teaspoon chopped garlic

1/3 cup (50 g) crumbled feta cheese

Throw your block of spinach in a microwaveable casserole with a lid, add a couple of tablespoons (28 ml) of water, and cover. Nuke it on high for 6 minutes.

In the meantime, chop your half an onion; I used my little food processor. Put your big, heavy skillet over a medium-low flame and start sautéing the onion.

If you didn't buy your pine nuts already toasted (very convenient!), put them in a little skillet, dry, over medium low heat; don't forget to stir them every couple of minutes or at least shake the skillet.

Okay, your microwave has beeped. Stir up the spinach. If your microwave is like mine, it won't be hot through yet. Break up what's left of the block and nuke for another 3 to 4 minutes. Go back to your skillets! You don't want anything to burn. If your onion's translucent, turn the heat off. Ditto if your pine nuts have a touch of gold.

When your spinach is done (but not overcooked, hot clear through will do), drain it quite well and stir it into the onion. Add the garlic and stir it in. Then stir in the feta. Serve with the toasted pine nuts on top.

Yield: 3 servings, each with 187 calories, 16 grams fat, 7 grams protein, 7 grams carbohydrate, 3 grams dietary fiber, and 4 grams usable carb.

⏲ Lemon-Mustard Asparagus

This is a simple variation of the traditional *Asparagus with Lemon Butter* in *500 Low-Carb Recipes*.

> 1 pound (455 g) asparagus
>
> 3 tablespoons (42 g) butter
>
> 1 1/2 teaspoons lemon juice
>
> 1 1/2 teaspoons spicy brown or Dijon mustard

Snap the ends off the asparagus spears where they break naturally. Put the asparagus in a microwaveable casserole or lay it flat in a glass pie plate. Add a couple of tablespoons (28 ml) of water, cover (use plastic wrap or a plate to cover a pie plate), and microwave on High for 3 to 4 minutes.

While the asparagus is cooking, melt the butter over low heat and stir in the lemon juice and mustard. (If you prefer, you can wait until the asparagus is cooked and melt the butter in the microwave, too.)

When the asparagus comes out of the microwave, uncover it right away or it will continue to cook and become gray and mushy within 5 minutes! Arrange on 4 serving plates and divide the lemon-mustard sauce between the servings.

Yield: 4 servings, each with 3 grams of carbohydrates and 1 gram of fiber, for a total of 2 grams of usable carbs and 2 grams of protein.

⊕ Asparagus with Soy and Sesame Mayonnaise

Serve this with fish for a fast and elegant company meal. It's super-easy to double or even triple.

  1 pound (455 g) asparagus

  1/2 cup (115 g) mayonnaise

  2 teaspoons soy sauce

  1 teaspoon dark sesame oil

  1 scallion

  1/4 teaspoon chili garlic sauce

Snap the ends off the asparagus where they want to break naturally. Put them in a microwave steamer or a Pyrex pie plate. Add a couple of tablespoons (28 ml) of water, cover, and nuke on high for 5 minutes.

In the meantime, assemble everything else in your food processor with the S-blade in place and run until the scallion is pulverized.

The standard way to serve this is to give everyone a puddle of sauce to dip their asparagus in. The fancy way is to spoon the sauce into a baggie, snip a teeny bit off the corner, and pipe artistic squiggles of sauce over your plates of asparagus.

By the way, if you nuke the asparagus earlier in the day and then chill it, this makes a nice salad.

Yield: 3 servings, each with 298 calories, 33 grams fat, 3 grams protein, 4 grams carbohydrate, 2 grams dietary fiber, and 2 grams usable carb.

⊕ Aparagus Parmesan

If you're paying really close attention, you'll notice that this is the asparagus from the *Asparagi All'uovo* (see page 52), without the eggs. It's a great side dish with a simple chicken breast.

    1 pound (455 g) asparagus
    1/2 teaspoon minced garlic or 1 clove garlic, crushed
    1/4 cup (60 ml) olive oil
    Salt and pepper
    1/2 cup (50 g) grated Parmesan cheese*

* Using good-quality cheese instead of the cheap stuff in the green shaker pays off here.

Snap the bottoms off the asparagus spears where they break naturally. Put the asparagus in a microwaveable casserole or a glass pie plate. Add a couple of tablespoons (28 ml) water, cover (use plastic wrap or a plate to cover a pie plate), and microwave on High for 3 to 4 minutes.

While the asparagus is cooking, stir the garlic into the olive oil.

When the asparagus is done, drain it. If you have 4 single-serving ovenproof dishes that are large enough to hold asparagus, they're ideal for this purpose—divide the asparagus between the 4 dishes. If not, you'll need to use a rectangular glass baking dish. Arrange the asparagus in 4 groups in the baking dish, like little stacks of cordwood.

Whether you're using the individual dishes or the single baking dish long enough to hold asparagus, drizzle each serving of asparagus with the garlic and olive oil. Salt and pepper lightly and divide the cheese between the servings. Put the asparagus under the broiler, about 4 inches (10 cm) from low heat. It'll need maybe 4 to 5 minutes. When the Parmesan cheese is touched with gold, serve.

Yield: 4 servings, each with 3 grams of carbohydrates and 1 gram of fiber, for a total of 2 grams of usable carbs and 6 grams of protein.

⊕ Simple Grilled Asparagus

Something about the grilling process accentuates the flavor of this dish.
Feel free to do this over your outdoor grill in the summer, by the way.

> 1 pound (455 g) asparagus
> 2 to 3 tablespoons (28 to 45 ml) olive oil
> Salt and pepper

Preheat your electric tabletop grill.

Snap the ends off the asparagus spears where they break naturally. Place the asparagus on a large plate, drizzle the olive oil over it, and then turn it all about with
clean hands, so each spear is coated with olive oil. Salt and pepper it.

Lay the asparagus on your grill. How much will fit at once will depend on
how big a grill you have; mine will fit most of a pound (455 g). Let it cook for
5 to 6 minutes and then serve.

Yield: 4 servings, each with 3 grams of carbohydrates and 1 gram of fiber,
for a total of 2 grams of usable carbs and 1 gram of protein.

⊕ Asparagus Bacon Bundles

This dish tastes great and has a cool-looking presentation, to boot!

>1 pound (455 g) pencil-thin asparagus
>
>7 slices bacon

Preheat your electric tabletop grill.

Snap the ends off the asparagus spears where they break naturally. Divide the asparagus into 7 bunches and wrap a slice of bacon in a spiral around each bunch. (In other words, don't let the bacon overlap itself, but cover as much of the asparagus bundle as you can.)

Place the asparagus-bacon bundles on the grill. How many will fit will depend on how big your grill is; mine will just fit all 7. Close the grill, let them cook for 7 minutes or until the bacon is done through, and serve.

Yield: 7 servings, each with 2 grams of carbohydrates and 1 gram of fiber, for a total of 1 gram of usable carbs and 3 grams of protein.

⊕ Blue Slaw

This is a really unusual twist on slaw.

>4 cups (360 g) bagged coleslaw mix
>
>3 tablespoons (45 g) plain yogurt
>
>1 tablespoon (15 g) sour cream
>
>1/4 cup (14 g) mayonnaise
>
>2 tablespoons (16 g) crumbled blue cheese

Just mix everything together—that's all!

Yield: 4 or 5 servings. Assuming 4 servings, each will have 5 grams of carbohydrates and 2 grams of fiber, for a total of 3 grams of usable carbs and 3 grams of protein.

Note: If you want, you can streamline this further by substituting 1/2 cup (115 g) bottled blue cheese dressing, but it's likely to have a little added sugar. Not much, but a little.

⊕ Hot and Sweet Mostly Asian Slaw

This is *mostly* Asian because of that hot wax pepper. You could use another mildly hot pepper in its place—an Anaheim, maybe, but that still wouldn't be Asian. It would still be good, though.

> 1 hot wax pepper (aka banana pepper)
>
> 1 medium carrot
>
> 1 bag (14 ounces, or 390 g) coleslaw mix
>
> 1/4 cup (4 g) minced cilantro
>
> 1/4 cup (60 ml) rice vinegar
>
> 1/4 cup (6 g) Splenda, or its equivalent in sweetness
>
> 1 tablespoon (15 ml) dark sesame oil

Split your pepper down the middle, remove the seeds, and slice it crosswise, very thin. Shred your carrot, too, and mince your cilantro. Throw them in a mixing bowl with the bagged coleslaw mix.

Mix together the vinegar, Splenda, and sesame oil and pour over the salad. Toss well and serve.

Yield: 4 servings, each with 73 calories, 4 grams fat, 2 grams protein, 10 grams carbohydrate, 3 grams dietary fiber, and 7 grams usable carb.

Note: Don't forget to wash your hands well after handling the pepper.

⊕ Orange Green Salad

This one's good with anything Mexican or Southwestern in flavor.

8 ounces (225 g) bagged mixed greens—I like half romaine,
half red leaf lettuce.

1/2 cup (8 g) chopped cilantro

1/4 sweet red onion, thinly sliced

2 tablespoons (28 ml) orange juice

2 tablespoons (28 ml) white wine vinegar

1/4 teaspoon minced garlic or 1/2 clove garlic, crushed

1/4 teaspoon ground cumin

4 tablespoons (60 ml) oil—A bland oil like canola or peanut is best for this.

Put the greens, cilantro, and onion in a large salad bowl. Mix together the juice, vinegar, garlic, and cumin and set it aside. Pour the oil over the salad and toss well until all the greens are coated. Pour in the orange juice mixture, toss again, and serve.

Yield: 4 servings, each with 6 grams of carbohydrates and 2 grams of fiber, for a total of 4 grams of usable carbs and 2 grams of protein.

⊕ Lime-Peanut Cucumber Salad

I just love cucumber salad, and I love peanuts in cucumber salad!

1/4 cup (35 g) dry-roasted peanuts

1/4 cup (40 g) red onion

1/4 cup (4 g) cilantro

1 large cucumber

1/4 cup (60 ml) lime juice

1/4 cup (60 ml) rice vinegar

1 teaspoon chopped garlic

1/4 teaspoon salt

1/4 teaspoon Sriracha chili sauce

2 teaspoons Splenda, or the equivalent in liquid Splenda

Put the peanuts in your food processor with the S-blade in place and pulse to chop. Dump them into a little bowl. Now put your onion and cilantro in the food processor and pulse to chop them. Dump those into a mixing bowl.

Swap the S-blade for the slicing blade. Quarter your cucumber lengthwise and run it through the slicing blade. Add it to the mixing bowl with the onion and cilantro.

Mix together the lime juice, rice vinegar, crushed garlic, salt, chili garlic paste, and Splenda and pour them over the salad. Toss well. Add the peanuts, toss again, and serve.

Yield: 4 servings, each with 79 calories, 5 grams fat, 3 grams protein, 8 grams carbohydrate, 2 grams dietary fiber, and 6 grams usable carb.

☺ Spinach Salad with Maple Glazed Bacon, Nectarines, and Feta

Even including making the salad dressing, I got this done by the 15 minute buzzer. This was inspired by a description I saw in my local paper of a salad made during a cooking contest by the best chef in town (David Tallent of Bloomington, Indiana). I just took the description and ran with it.

> 4 bacon slices
>
> 1/4 cup (80 g) sugar-free pancake syrup
>
> 6 cups (180 g) baby spinach leaves
>
> 1/2 nectarine (You could use a peach, but you'd have to peel it, which takes another minute or two.)
>
> 1/4 cup (75 g) crumbled feta cheese
>
> 1/4 small red onion, sliced paper-thin
>
> *Maple-Bacon Vinaigrette* (See recipe on page 301.)

First let's take care of the bacon: Brush it both sides with the pancake syrup and lay it on a microwave bacon rack or in a Pyrex pie plate. Nuke it on high for 7 or 8 minutes—for some reason glazed bacon takes longer; go figure.

Now make your *Maple-Bacon Vinaigrette*. (See page 301 for the recipe.)

After that, dice your half of a nectarine and if you didn't buy your feta already crumbled, crumble it.

Pile your spinach in a big salad bowl. Pour on the dressing and toss until it's evenly coated. Top with the nectarine and feta and snip your now-crisp glazed bacon over the top. Fall face first into the salad bowl. No, I mean pile it on 3 or 4 salad plates and serve!

Yield: 3 to 4 servings, assuming 3, each will have 287 calories, 25 grams fat, 7 grams protein, 9 grams carbohydrate, 2 grams dietary fiber, and 7 grams usable carb.

⊕ Red Leaf Lettuce with Melon and Feta

What a beautiful summer salad this is! It could be a main dish salad, too, if you shared it between just two.

> 7 1/2 cups (210 g) red leaf lettuce, torn up
>
> 4 tablespoons (60 ml) vinaigrette—I like Newman's Own Olive Oil and Vinegar.
>
> 2/3 cup (100 g) crumbled feta cheese
>
> 1/2 yellow bell pepper, diced
>
> 2/3 cup (107 g) purchased cantaloupe cubes
>
> 2 tablespoons (18 g) roasted, salted sunflower seed kernels

Put lettuce in a big salad bowl, add vinaigrette, and toss. Add the feta and toss again. Pile on plates, top with the other ingredients, and serve.

Yield: 4 servings, each with 199 calories, 17 grams fat, 6 grams protein, 8 grams carbohydrate, 2 grams dietary fiber, and 6 grams usable carb.

⊕ Gorgonzola and Pesto Caesar Salad

Oh, all right, use another blue cheese if you must. But being Italian and all, gorgonzola is best here.

> 6 cups (282 g) romaine lettuce hearts, broken up
>
> 3 tablespoons (45 ml) extra virgin olive oil
>
> 1 1/2 tablespoons (23 g) pesto sauce
>
> 1/3 cup (40 g) crumbled gorgonzola cheese

This is super simple! Put your lettuce in a big salad bowl. Mix the olive oil and pesto together and then pour over salad and toss furiously until it's all evenly coated. Sprinkle the gorgonzola over the whole thing, toss lightly again, and serve.

Yield: 4 servings, each with 163 calories, 16 grams fat, 4 grams protein, 3 grams carbohydrate, 2 grams dietary fiber, and 1 gram usable carb.

⊕ Quick Winter Salad

This is so good! It's like Waldorf salad brought into the 21st century. This keeps very well in a snap-top container in the fridge, and it is a great choice for a potluck or if you want to make something special ahead of time.

 1/4 cup (34 g) shelled hazelnuts

 2 large celery ribs

 1 fennel bulb

 1 apple—I used a Gala, and it was great.

 1/3 cup (80 ml) olive oil

 2 tablespoons (22 g) brown mustard

 2 tablespoons (28 ml) white vinegar

 1 tablespoon (15 ml) lemon juice

 1/4 teaspoon salt or Vege-Sal

 1/2 teaspoon chopped garlic

 1/4 cup (25 g) grated Parmesan cheese

Put the hazelnuts in a Pyrex pie plate and microwave on high for 2 minutes or until fragrant—give them a 3rd minute if they need it.

While your hazelnuts are toasting, run your celery and fennel through the slicing blade of your food processor. Cut your apple into matchstick strips; unless you have a julienne blade you'll have to do this by hand. (The easiest way I've found to do this is to quarter it, remove the core, and then set each quarter, in turn, on your cutting board. Cut straight down through the quarter, lengthwise—in other words, don't cut it into thin wedges, just evenly thick slices. Then cut across those to make matchstick strips.) Throw all your veggies in a big salad bowl.

By now the microwave has beeped. Pull your hazelnuts out and let them cool a few minutes.

Measure the olive oil, mustard, vinegar, lemon juice, and salt or Vege-Sal. Crush the garlic and throw it in, too. Whisk everything together well and pour it over the salad. Toss until everything's evenly coated.

Yield: 5 servings, each with 231 calories, 21 grams fat, 4 grams protein, 11 grams carbohydrate, 3 grams fiber, and 8 grams usable carbs.

☺ Vegetables Vinaigrette

If your grocery store carries frozen mixed stir-fry peppers with onions, they're a handy item to have in the house. This is gorgeous—and tasty, too. A great choice for a dinner party.

> 1 pound (455 g) asparagus
>
> 3 tablespoons (45 ml) olive oil
>
> 1 bag (1 pound, or 455 g) frozen mixed stir-fry peppers with onions, thawed
>
> 1/3 cup (80 ml) Italian vinaigrette dressing

Snap the ends off of the asparagus spears where they break naturally. Slice them diagonally into 1/2-inch (1.3 cm) lengths.

Heat the oil in a large, heavy skillet or wok over high heat. Add the asparagus and stir-fry for 1 to 2 minutes. Add the peppers, and continue stir-frying until the vegetables are tender-crisp. Stir in the dressing, let the whole thing cook for another minute, and serve.

Yield: 6 to 8 servings. Assuming 8 servings, each will have 7 grams of carbohydrates and 2 grams of fiber, for a total of 5 grams of usable carbs and 1 gram of protein.

☺ Orange Pecan Sprouts

My husband took a bite of these, pointed to his plate, and said, "You could make these again!" They are really wonderful.

 1 pound (455 g) brussels sprouts

 1/3 cup (37 g) chopped pecans

 3 tablespoons (42 g) butter

 1 teaspoon grated orange zest

 3 tablespoons (45 ml) orange juice

Trim the stems of the brussels sprouts and remove any wilted outer leaves. Run the sprouts through the slicing blade of your food processor.

In a large, heavy skillet over medium-high heat, start sautéing the pecans in the butter. After about 2 minutes, add the brussels sprouts and sauté the two together, stirring every few minutes, until the sprouts soften and start to have a few brown spots. While they're sautéing, you can grate the orange zest and squeeze the orange juice. (You could use bottled orange juice, but since you need the zest, too, fresh just makes sense.) When the sprouts are tender and flecked with brown, stir in the zest and juice, cook for just another minute, and serve.

Yield: 4 servings, each with 12 grams of carbohydrates and 5 grams of fiber, for a total of 7 grams of usable carbs and 4 grams of protein.

☉Brussels and Bacon

My husband and I thought we didn't like brussels sprouts. Turned out we'd only had them boiled and buttered—and that's the only way we don't like them. Once we tried them fried, it was a quick jump to sautéed, roasted, and grilled, and we loved them every way we tried them. So if you think you don't like brussels sprouts, think again!

> 2 bacon slices
>
> 1 pound (455 g) brussels sprouts
>
> salt and pepper

Put your big, heavy skillet over medium-low heat and snip the bacon into it in pieces no wider than 1/4 inch (6 mm). Let that cook.

Trim the very bottoms of the brussels sprouts and remove any really ugly leaves. Now go stir your bacon.

Run your brussels sprouts through the slicing blade of your food processor. By now your bacon should be getting browned. Dump the sliced brussels sprouts in with the bacon and stir it all up. Cover the skillet and turn the burner up just a smidge.

Let the brussels sprouts cook for the remainder of your fifteen minutes, stirring every couple of minutes and then re-covering. Salt, pepper, and serve!

Yield: 3 to 4 servings, assuming 4, each will have 62 calories, 2 grams fat, 4 grams protein, 9 grams carbohydrate, 4 grams dietary fiber, and 5 grams usable carb.

⊕Mustardy Grilled Brussels

This recipe really requires frozen, thawed brussels sprouts—they cook faster than fresh ones.

> 1/4 cup (60 ml) olive oil
>
> 2 tablespoons (22 g) brown mustard
>
> 1/4 teaspoon pepper, or to taste
>
> 1 pound (455 g) frozen brussels sprouts, thawed
>
> salt

Preheat your electric tabletop grill to its highest temperature; I set mine for 425°F (220°C).

Measure the olive oil, mustard, and pepper into a mixing bowl and whisk them together. Dump in the brussels sprouts and stir to coat.

Arrange your brussels sprouts on your grill—I have the big size George Foreman grill with the snap-out grill plates, and it fit a pound of brussels sprouts handily.

Set a timer for 10 minutes—longer if your grill doesn't get quite so hot. You want your brussels sprouts good and dark brown, nearly burnt, where they touch the grill plates.

When they come off the grill—use a pair of tongs—you can serve them just salted, which is very nice. Or you can put them back in the mixing bowl, toss them with the residual oil and mustard mixture, and then serve. They're super either way.

Yield: 3 to 4 servings, assuming 3, each will have 231 calories, 19 grams fat, 6 grams protein, 13 grams carbohydrate, 6 grams dietary fiber, and 7 grams usable carb.

⊕ Super Simple Grilled Eggplant

I really worked at getting a simple, quick eggplant recipe in here. This was my best try, but how many servings you can make and how quickly will depend on the size of your electric tabletop grill and how hot it will get. I have a good, big one with adjustable heat. Not to mention that it has grill plates that snap out and go in the dishwasher, which is a fine thing.

>   1 medium eggplant, whole
>   1 cup (235 ml) olive oil

Start your electric tabletop grill heating to its highest setting; I used 425°F (220°C).

Pour the olive oil into a large, flat pan.

Slice your eggplant crosswise, about 1 inch (2.5 cm) thick. As you cut each slice, drop it in the olive oil. Keep slicing and after a few seconds, flip the ones already in the oil. When they're nice and oily both sides, put them on the grill and throw some more eggplant in the oil. You may need more oil; eggplant is like a sponge.

Grill the eggplant until it's a nice brown; I like it pretty well done, maybe 7 to 8 minutes. I can fit 6 slices on my grill at a time; figure that's three servings. I got 4 to 5 servings all told, but the second batch came in past the 15 minute mark. So this is a 15 minute recipe for three or for 6 who only want once slice of eggplant!

Just salt and pepper and eat it. It's yummy.

Yield: 4 servings, each with 507 calories, 54 grams fat, 1 grams protein, 7 grams carbohydrate, 3 grams dietary fiber, and 4 grams usable carb.

⊕ Cumin Mushrooms

This is a simply amazing accompaniment to the *Many-Pepper Steak* (see page 141). It's also a killer omelet filling (see page 35).

8 ounces (225 g) sliced mushrooms

1 1/2 tablespoons (21 g) butter

1 1/2 tablespoons (23 ml) olive oil

1 teaspoon ground cumin

1/4 teaspoon pepper

2 tablespoons (30 g) sour cream

Start sautéing the mushrooms in the butter and oil over medium-high heat. When they've gone limp and changed color, stir in the cumin and pepper. Let the mushrooms cook with the spices for a minute or two, stir in the sour cream, cook just long enough to heat through, and serve.

Yield: 3 or 4 servings. Assuming 3 servings, each will have 4 grams of carbohydrates and 1 gram of fiber, for a total of 3 grams of usable carbs and 2 grams of protein.

⊕Mushrooms with Bacon, Sun-Dried Tomatoes, and Cheese

Just looking at the ingredients in the title, you know you'll love this!

4 slices bacon

8 ounces (225 g) sliced mushrooms

1/2 teaspoon minced garlic or 1 clove fresh garlic

1/4 cup (14 g) diced sun-dried tomatoes—about 10 pieces before dicing

2 tablespoons (28 ml) heavy cream

1/3 cup (27 g) shredded Parmesan cheese

Chop up the bacon or snip it up with kitchen shears. Start cooking it in a large, heavy skillet over medium-high heat. As some grease starts to cook out of the bacon, stir in the mushrooms.

Let the mushrooms cook until they start to change color and get soft. Stir in the garlic and cook for 4 to 5 more minutes. Stir in the tomatoes and cream and cook until the cream is absorbed. Scatter the cheese over the whole thing, stir it in, let it cook for just another minute, and serve.

Yield: 3 or 4 servings. Assuming 4 servings, each will have 5 grams of carbohydrates and 1 gram of fiber, for a total of 4 grams of usable carbs and 6 grams of protein.

☺Mushrooms Au Gratin

This is just fantastic with a steak, and try the leftovers in an omelet! Nearly any shredded cheese would be good here, so feel free to experiment.

16 ounces (455 g) sliced mushrooms—Buy them that way!

3 tablespoons (42 g) butter

2 egg yolks

1/3 cup (77 g) sour cream

1/4 teaspoon salt or Vege-Sal

1/4 teaspoon pepper

1/2 cup (58 g) shredded Monterey Jack cheese—or swiss, mexican blend, etc.

In your big, heavy skillet, over medium-high heat, start the mushrooms cooking in the butter. Cover with a tilted lid.

In the meantime, separate your eggs and find something constructive to do with the whites. Stir your mushrooms and re-cover. Put the yolks in a bowl, add the sour cream, add the salt or Vege-Sal and pepper, and whisk it all together until smooth. Go stir your mushrooms and again re-cover.

When the mushrooms have all softened and changed color a bit, turn the burner to lowest heat and stir in the sour cream mixture. Sprinkle the cheese evenly over all, re-cover, and let it cook until the fifteen minutes is up and the cheese is melted; then serve.

Yield: 4 to 5 servings, assuming 4, each will have 228 calories, 20 grams fat, 8 grams protein, 6 grams carbohydrate, 1 gram dietary fiber, and 5 grams usable carb.

⏱ Cheese and Chipotle Portobellos

I wasn't sure where to put these! They'd make a fine appetizer, a great side dish, or you could even serve two apiece as a light entree.

>   6 tablespoons (84 g) mayonnaise
>
>   2 chipotle chiles canned in adobo
>
>   6 Portobello mushroom caps
>
>   6 ounces (170 g) Swiss cheese in 6 slices

Preheat your electric tabletop grill to 350°F (180°C).

Run the chilies and mayo through your food processor. Brush the convex sides of the mushroom caps with a little of the chipotle mayo and then fill the cavities with a spoonful of the mayo. Put them in the grill filled-side up. Set a timer for 5 minutes.

When the timer beeps, open the grill and cover each mushroom with Swiss cheese—if the slices are bigger than the mushroom caps, tear and overlap them to fit. Use a cup or jar to prop the grill lid just far enough open that it's not touching the cheese and give the mushrooms another minute to 90 seconds—just long enough to melt the cheese.

Plate the mushrooms, spoon the rest of the chipotle mayo on top, and serve.

Yield: 6 servings, each with 237 calories, 20 grams fat, 11 grams protein, 7 grams carbohydrate, 2 grams dietary fiber, and 5 grams usable carb.

⊕ Briar Rose's Artichoke Salad

A cyberpal with the screen name Briar Rose suggested this combination of ingredients to me, and it sounded so phenomenal I just had to play with it. Extraordinary! I was hard-pressed to know whether to call this a side dish or a main dish salad—it's in the in-between range, protein-wise. Call it a substantial side dish or a light meal.

> 1 can (13.75 ounces, or 385 g) quartered artichoke hearts,
>   drained and coarsely chopped
> 2 ounces (55 g) sliced pepperoni, sliced into 1/4-inch (6mm) strips
> 1/4 cup (40 g) chopped sweet red onion*
> 2 tablespoons (6 g) chopped fresh basil
> 1/2 cup (60 g) crumbled Gorgonzola
> 3 tablespoons (45 ml) extra-virgin olive oil
> 1/2 teaspoon minced garlic or 1 clove garlic, crushed
> 1 1/2 tablespoons (23 ml) balsamic vinegar

* Actually, Briar Rose doesn't like this, so leave it out if you want to. I'm hopelessly devoted to red onion.

Simply mix everything together and stir well. That's it!

I like to serve this on a bed of lettuce, but it's remarkably good right out of the mixing bowl. For that matter, you could toss it with lettuce that's been broken up well or with bagged mixed greens. Oh, heck, it's hard to think of a bad way to serve this!

Yield: 3 servings, each with 11 grams of carbohydrates and 1 gram of fiber, for a total of 10 grams of usable carbs (though quite a lot of that is a carbohydrate called "inulin," found in artichokes, which has the lowest blood sugar impact of any carbohydrate yet identified, so this is actually a lot easier on your body than the carb count suggests) and 11 grams of protein.

Tip: To save time, stack up the pepperoni rounds and slice them several at a time.

Note: Gorgonzola is the Italian version of blue cheese (although the veins are actually greenish). It's a little milder and creamier than a lot of blue cheeses, and it's quite delicious. However, if you can't find Gorgonzola, feel free to substitute your favorite blue cheese.

⊕ Country-Style Green Beans

Okay, truly country-style green beans are cooked for a billion hours with bacon or a ham hock, but that hardly makes for a 15-minute recipe, now does it? And this version tastes very good and down-home.

> 1 pound (455 g) frozen cut green beans
>
> 3 slices bacon
>
> 4 ounces (115 g) sliced mushrooms
>
> 1/2 tablespoon butter
>
> 1 tablespoon (15 ml) lemon juice

Put the beans in a microwaveable casserole with a lid, add a couple of tablespoons (28 ml) of water, cover, and microwave on High for 7 minutes.

Cut the bacon into little pieces and put it in a large, heavy skillet—I use kitchen shears to snip it right into the pan—and start cooking it over medium-high heat. When a little grease starts to cook out of the bacon, add the mushrooms and butter and cook it all together, stirring frequently, until the bacon is starting to get crispy and the mushrooms have softened and changed color.

Somewhere during this process, your microwave is going to go "ding!" When it does, go check the beans. Chances are they'll still be underdone in the center, so stir them up and give them another 4 to 5 minutes.

When the beans are tender-crisp, pull them out of the microwave, drain them, and stir them into the bacon and mushrooms. Stir in the lemon juice, let the whole thing cook together for just another minute or two to combine the flavors, and then serve.

Yield: 4 or 5 servings. Assuming 4 servings, each will have 10 grams of carbohydrates and 4 grams of fiber, for a total of 6 grams of usable carbs and 4 grams of protein.

⊕ Hazelnut Green Beans

Do you love Green Beans Almandine? Try these for a change.

1 pound (455 g) frozen green beans

¼ cup (34 g) hazelnuts

2 tablespoons (28 ml) olive oil

2 tablespoons (28 ml) lemon juice

salt and pepper

Put your green beans in a microwaveable casserole with a lid, add a couple of tablespoons (28 ml) of water, and nuke on high for 7 minutes.

In the meantime, chop your hazelnuts. Put your big, heavy skillet over medium heat, add the olive oil, and sauté the hazelnuts until they're touched with gold and smell wonderful. Remove from the heat.

By now the microwave has beeped. Go stir your beans and give them another 3 or 4 minutes.

When your beans are tender-crisp, drain and add to the skillet along with the lemon juice. Toss everything together, salt and pepper to taste, and serve.

Yield: 4 servings, each with 154 calories, 12 grams fat, 3 grams protein, 11 grams carbohydrate, 4 grams dietary fiber, and 7 grams usable carb.

Regarding Bagged Salad

There are now approximately 482 varieties of bagged salad available in your average grocery store, and what a fine development that is. For once we have a packaged food that is as good for us as it is convenient, sing Glory Hallelujah!

Do yourself a favor and venture beyond the standard Iceberg Mix or American Blend. Iceberg is the least nutritious of the lettuces and the blandest, as well. If you buy bagged salad, try a new blend at least once every couple of weeks, to find out what you might have been missing.

You'll probably be buying bottled salad dressing, too. Remember that the fat-free dressings virtually always have a lot of added sugar! So, too, does any dressing that tastes sweet—Russian, Catalina, that red stuff that calls itself "French," Poppyseed, Honey Mustard, Raspberry Vinaigrette. All are likely culprits, so read the labels carefully.

Overall, you can trust most of the following dressings in their full-fat versions: Blue Cheese (occasionally called Roquefort), Caesar, Creamy Garlic, Red Wine Vinaigrette, Italian, Ranch, Parmesan Peppercorn. However, read the labels to find the brands with the lowest sugar content.

Here's an unsolicited plug: I love Paul Newman's salad dressings. At this writing, I have his Original Olive Oil and Vinegar, Caesar, and Balsamic Vinaigrette in the house, and I think they're all terrific. If you buy the full-fat versions of Paul's dressings they tend to be lower carb than similar dressings in other brands, and they contain no junk chemicals. It's good stuff; look for them.

Now, bagged greens with bottled dressings are all well and good, but sometimes you want something more in your salads. I trust you're clear on the idea of adding some diced green pepper, sliced cucumber, some sliced scallions or sweet onion, a radish or two, or a few cherry tomatoes, but what if you want some crunch to replace the croutons? Try the following:

Sunflower seeds.

Diced or broken pork rinds.

Sliced, toasted, flavored almonds. Sunkist recently started distributing these under the name "Almond Accents." They're very crisp and tasty, and they come in a neat variety of flavors, including Roasted Garlic Caesar, Italian Parmesan, Bacon Cheddar, Garlic Teriyaki, Ranch, and Nacho Cheese. Look for them in the produce aisle of big grocery stores. These make a nice snack, too.

Crumbled bacon. I can't abide fake bacon bits, nor do I like the real bacon bits in a jar—they're soggy and flat-tasting, if you ask me. But it's not much work to throw a few slices of bacon into a glass pie plate, microwave them on High for a few minutes, and then crumble them up. (In most microwaves, about 1 minute per slice is about right, but you'll have to play with your microwave to know for sure.)

Crunchy cheesy bits. If you're used to putting shredded cheddar or the like on your salads, try this: Spray a microwaveable plate with nonstick cooking spray and throw a good handful of cheese—cheddar, Monterey Jack, Parmesan, or any natural, unprocessed hard cheese—on it. Use maybe 1/3 to 1/2 cup (38 to 58 g). Microwave on High for 1 minute. (The time may vary a bit, depending on your microwave.) It will melt into a disc that will be crispy as it cools. Crumble it over your salad for crunchy, crouton-like bits that have all the full flavor of cheese! This also makes a great snack.

Another thing to consider on busy nights is foregoing salad in favor of cut-up vegetables with dip. One real benefit of this is that—according to my sister Kim, The World's Best Second Grade Teacher—children will eat virtually anything if you give them Ranch dressing to dip it in. Put out a plate of celery sticks, pepper strips, cut-up broccoli and cauliflower, and some baby carrots (which you'll go easy on, right?), along with a bowl of Ranch dressing while you're getting the rest of the meal on the table. You know—do this while the family is starved and looking for something to eat right now. You may be surprised how many vegetables you can get into them this way (especially if you hide the chips) and with almost no work.

Regarding the Virtues of the Salad Bar

Salad bars aren't as common in grocery stores as they were 10 to 12 years back, which is a darn shame—but you can still find grocery stores that have these exceedingly useful features. If you're a reluctant cook, it is worth your while to seek out a local grocery store that does have a salad bar.

Why? Well, obviously it will let you make salads easily. But more than that, it's a great source of prepared ingredients. Do you use chopped onions a lot? Buy a container of pre-chopped onions from the salad bar, enough for 3 or 4 days, and stash 'em in the fridge. Do you need sliced peppers for a stir-fry? Hit the salad bar! Heck, I remember being at the salad bar at Sunset Foods in Highland Park, Illinois, on the day before Thanksgiving many years ago, and watching all the local women buying the onions and celery and such for their turkey stuffing. I was dumbstruck with admiration for their cleverness.

So check out the local salad bar and see what pre-prepped ingredients it offers you!

Regarding Plain Cooked Vegetables

When you're in a hurry and in the mood for a simple, plain cooked vegetable, you have a couple of choices. Fresh vegetables, although wonderful, will generally be the most work, although you can find some of them (most notably broccoli and cauliflower) cut up and ready to cook in your grocery store's produce section. But if you're trying to do minimal cooking, you probably won't want to take the time to, say, top and tail a whole pound (455 g) of green beans or trim the stems and leaves of several dozen Brussels sprouts.

This leaves you with canned or frozen. Personally, I much prefer frozen vegetables. I consider them superior to canned both in taste and texture, not to mention nutrition. (The canned-good manufacturers insist that canned vegetables are just as good, nutritionally, as frozen or fresh. This is apparently so—provided you consume all the water in the can, and who ever does that, except when making soup?) I'd go with the frozen vegetables, of which your grocery store freezer section has an ever-expanding variety.

The most important thing to know about frozen vegetables is the fastest, easiest way to cook them to get superior results, both for eating quality and nutrition. That method is microwaving. You've probably noticed the repeated use of the microwave in the recipes here. This is because the microwave is one of the very best ways to cook vegetables, yielding results that are better than boiling or steaming vegetables on the stove, and—because very little water is used—retaining more vitamins, too. Almost all frozen vegetables now come with microwave instructions on the package. Use them!

Another important tip: No matter what method you use to cook your vegetables, when they are done to your taste, uncover them. Do not keep the lid on them while you finish preparing the rest of the meal. I know you're just trying to keep them warm, but what you're actually doing is letting them continue cooking. That's how they end up gray and mushy and icky, and your kids grow up hating vegetables. Better to remove the lid to let out the steam, and then—if the rest of dinner is going to take another 5 to 10 minutes—put the lid back on, leaving a 1/2-inch (1.3 cm) crack. This will hold in heat without overcooking your veggies. If the meal is seriously delayed, you can always reheat your vegetables for a minute or two, which is a lot better than cooking them to a pulp.

You'll serve your veggies with butter and a little salt and pepper, no doubt, but don't forget that there are easy things to do with vegetables, too. A little lemon juice is wonderful on many vegetables, especially broccoli and green beans. Garlic is good, too, and you can buy garlic-infused olive oil to drizzle over vegetables to great effect. (You can also make your own by putting a few cloves of crushed garlic or a few teaspoons of jarred, minced garlic in a squeeze bottle and filling it with olive oil.) Lemon-pepper is good on many veggies, and how about Cajun seasoning? It doesn't take a lot of work to do something a little different and good; it just takes remembering to do it.

15~Minute Soups

Of course, to keep within our 15-minute time limit, we won't be making slow-simmered soups. But I think you'll be surprised at just how good a soup you can make in so little time. One word of advice: Do buy the best-quality canned or boxed broth you can get. It makes a big difference.

☉ Cream of Salmon Soup

One person who sampled this soup pronounced it the best soup they'd ever had. And it's so easy!

> 1 1/2 tablespoons (21 g) butter
> 1/4 cup (40 g) finely minced onion
> 1/4 cup (25 g) finely minced celery
> 2 cups (475 ml) heavy cream
> 1 can (14 ounces, or 410 g) salmon, drained
> 1/2 teaspoon dried thyme

In a heavy saucepan, melt the butter over medium-low heat and add the onion and celery. Sauté the vegetables for a few minutes until the onion is turning translucent.

Meanwhile, pour the cream into a glass 2-cup (475 ml) measure or any other micro-wavable container big enough for it and from which you can pour. Place it in the microwave and heat it at 50 percent power for 3 to 4 minutes. (This just cuts the time needed to heat the cream through—you can skip this step and simply heat the soup on the stove top a little longer, if you like.)

Pour the cream into the saucepan and add the salmon and thyme. Break up the salmon as you stir the soup—I found my whisk to be ideal for breaking the salmon into fine pieces. Heat until simmering and serve.

Yield: 4 servings, each with 5 grams of carbohydrates, a trace of fiber, and 23 grams of protein.

⊕ Mexican Cabbage Soup

This is great on a nasty, cold, rainy night! This is not hot, despite the chilies in the canned tomatoes—feel free to pass the hot sauce at the table if you want to spice it up. With all these vegetables, this is a complete meal, but if the family insists, you could add some corn tortillas for them.

> 1 quart (950 ml) beef broth
>
> 1 can (14 ounces, or 410 g) diced tomatoes with green chilies
>
> 1 pound (455 g) ground round or other very lean ground beef
>
> 1 tablespoon (15 ml) oil
>
> 1/2 cup (80 g) chopped onion
>
> 1 teaspoon minced garlic or 2 cloves garlic, crushed
>
> 1 teaspoon ground cumin
>
> 2 teaspoons oregano
>
> 2 cups (180 g) bagged coleslaw mix

In a large, microwaveable container combine the beef broth and canned tomatoes. Microwave on High for 8 to 10 minutes.

While the broth and tomatoes are heating through, start browning and crumbling the beef in the oil. Use a large soup kettle or heavy-bottomed saucepan. When the beef's about half browned, add the onion and garlic. Continue cooking until the beef is entirely browned. Add the cumin and oregano, stir them in, and then add the heated beef stock and tomatoes. Stir in the coleslaw mix and bring the whole thing to a simmer. Cook for another minute or so and serve.

Yield: 4 servings, each with 9 grams of carbohydrates and 2 grams of fiber, for a total of 7 grams of usable carbs and 24 grams of protein.

⊕ Oyster Stew

This is a classic recipe that simply started out fast, easy, and low-carb. My husband prefers me to cut really big oysters into quarters. Since you can do this as the cream and half-and-half are heating, it doesn't add any time to the recipe—indeed, since the pieces of oyster cook faster than whole ones, it cuts the cooking time a bit.

> 5 tablespoons (70 g) butter
>
> 1 cup (235 ml) half-and-half
>
> 1 1/2 cups (355 ml) heavy cream
>
> 1/2 cup (120 ml) water
>
> 1 1/2 pints (680 g) oysters
>
> Salt and pepper
>
> 1/8 teaspoon cayenne

Put the butter, half-and-half, heavy cream, and water in a heavy-bottomed saucepan over medium heat. As it comes to a simmer, add the oysters and stir. Simmer until the oysters are cooked, about 5 minutes. Salt and pepper to taste, add the cayenne, and then serve.

Yield: 4 servings, each with 8 grams of carbohydrates, no fiber, and 11 grams of protein. Despite the modest protein count, this is filling because it is so rich.

Note: If you'd like to speed this recipe up, you can combine everything but the oysters in a good-size microwaveable container and nuke it for 5 minutes on High, but it's not essential.

☺ Stir-Fry Soup

The name says it all—a traditional stir-fry turned into a hearty soup. This works equally well with chicken or pork, so take your pick or use whatever is cluttering up the freezer.

> 2 quarts (1.9 L) chicken broth
>
> 1 pound (455 g) boneless pork loin or 1 pound (455 g) boneless, skinless chicken breast
>
> 1 medium onion
>
> 3 tablespoons (45 ml) oil
>
> 1 bag (16 ounces, or 455 g) frozen stir-fry vegetables, thawed
>
> 1 1/2 tablespoons (23 ml) soy sauce
>
> 1 1/2 tablespoons (23 ml) dry sherry
>
> 1 1/2 tablespoons (12 g) grated gingerroot
>
> 1 1/2 teaspoons minced garlic
>
> 1 1/2 teaspoons toasted sesame oil

Pour the chicken broth into a large microwaveable bowl or pitcher. Put it in the microwave and nuke it for 10 minutes on High.

Slice the pork or chicken as thin as possible. (This is easier if the meat is partly frozen.) Thinly slice the onion, as well. Heat the oil in the bottom of a large soup kettle and add the meat, onion, and stir-fry vegetables. Stir-fry everything over highest heat while the broth is warming in the microwave.

By the time the microwave goes "ding," the pork or chicken should not be pink anymore. Pour in the broth, add the soy sauce, sherry, gingerroot, garlic, and sesame oil, cover, and let the whole thing simmer for 4 to 5 minutes before serving.

Yield: 6 servings, each with 9 grams of carbohydrates and 2 grams of fiber, for a total of 7 grams of usable carbs and 19 grams of protein.

☉ Italian Sausage Soup

This takes some serious multi-tasking to get done in 15 minutes, but it was too good not to include.

1 1/2 quarts (1.4 L) chicken broth

1 bag (16 ounces, or 455 g) frozen Italian Vegetable Blend

1 pound (455 g) Italian sausage, mild or hot, as you prefer

1/2 medium onion, chopped

1 teaspoon minced garlic or 2 cloves garlic, crushed

2 teaspoons Italian seasoning

3 eggs

5 tablespoons (25 g) grated or shredded Parmesan cheese

First, put the broth in a good-size saucepan, cover it, and place it over high heat. Next, put the Italian Vegetable Blend in a microwaveable casserole, add a couple of tablespoons (28 ml) of water, cover, and microwave on High for 12 minutes.

Okay, that stuff is under control. Now, in a heavy-bottomed kettle, start browning the Italian sausage over medium-high heat. If the sausage is in links, slit the skins and squeeze it out, so you can crumble it; bulk sausage you can just plunk into the kettle. As a bit of grease starts to cook out of the sausage, add the onion and the garlic (you can chop the onion while the sausage is browning) and let them sauté together.

When the sausage is cooked through, add the chicken broth, which should be hot by now. Stir and add the Italian seasoning. Let the mixture simmer while you crack the eggs into a glass measuring cup and beat them with a fork. Pour the eggs in, a little bit at a time—pour, then stir, pour some more, and then stir some more. This will make lovely egg shreds in your soup.

The vegetables should be done by now, so pull them out of the microwave, drain, and dump them into the soup. Stir, let the whole thing simmer for just another minute, and serve with a tablespoon (5 g) of Parmesan cheese on each serving.

Yield: 5 servings, each with 11 grams of carbohydrates and 2 grams of fiber, for a total of 9 grams of usable carbs and 26 grams of protein.

⊕ Pantry Seafood Bisque

This recipe is quick, easy, tasty, and what a gorgeous pale pink color! It's simple to double, of course, but it'll take a little longer for the larger quantity of half-and-half to heat through. You could microwave it to speed things along, if you like.

1 pint (475 ml) half-and-half

3 tablespoons (48 g) tomato paste

1 can (4 ounces, or 115 g) tiny shrimp, drained

1 can (6 ounces, or 170 g) flaked crab, drained

1 teaspoon dried dill weed

1/2 teaspoon lemon juice

Salt and pepper to taste

In a largish saucepan over low heat, heat the half-and-half to just below a simmer. Whisk in the tomato paste and then stir in the shrimp, crab, dill, and lemon juice. Let the whole thing cook together for just a minute or two, salt and pepper to taste, and serve.

Yield: 3 servings, each with 11 grams of carbohydrates and 1 gram of fiber, for a total of 10 grams of usable carbs and 24 grams of protein.

☆ Each serving also has 254 milligrams of calcium!

☺ Almost Lobster Bisque

Monkfish has long been known as "poor man's lobster," so I decided to use it in a classic lobster bisque. However, if your budget allows, feel free to use lobster tail in this recipe instead.

1/2 cup (120 ml) heavy cream

1 cup (235 ml) half-and-half

1/2 cup (120 ml) water

10 ounce (280 g) monkfish fillet

1/2 cup (120 ml) dry sherry

1 1/2 teaspoons *Dana's No-Sugar Ketchup* (see page 309)
    or other sugar-free ketchup

1/2 teaspoon Worcestershire sauce

1/2 teaspoon lemon juice

1/2 teaspoon salt or Vege-Sal

Guar or xanthan (optional)

1 scallion, finely sliced

First combine the cream, half-and-half, and water in a large, microwaveable dish. Microwave for 5 to 6 minutes on 70 percent power.

While the cream is heating, cut the monkfish fillet into bite-size pieces. Bring the sherry to a simmer in a large, heavy-bottomed saucepan over medium-high heat. Add the monkfish, turn the burner down a touch, and let the fish simmer in the sherry, stirring occasionally, for 4 to 5 minutes or until cooked through.

Stir in the cream, which should be hot by now. Stir in the ketchup, Worcestershire sauce, lemon juice, and salt and heat it only to a simmer. If you'd like your bisque thicker, feel free to use guar or xanthan, but it's mighty nice the way it is. Ladle into dishes and top each serving with a scattering of sliced scallion.

Yield: 2 servings, each with 10 grams of carbohydrates, a trace of fiber, and 26 grams of protein.

⊕ Instant Chicken Soup

Okay, so this isn't quite as instant as those little packets you mix with boiling water. But it's a lot tastier, a lot heartier, and a lot better for you.

> ¹/₄ head cauliflower
>
> 1 quart (905 ml), or 2 cans (14.5 ounces, or 410 g) chicken broth
>
> 10 to 12 ounces (280 to 340 g) boneless, skinless chicken breast
>
> 1 stalk celery
>
> 1 medium carrot
>
> ¹/₄ medium onion
>
> 1 tablespoon (14 g) butter
>
> 1 ¹/₂ teaspoons poultry seasoning
>
> Salt and pepper

Run the cauliflower through the shredding blade of your food processor. Put it in a microwaveable bowl, add a tablespoon (15 ml) of water, cover, and microwave on High for 5 minutes.

While that's cooking, pour the broth into a large saucepan over high heat. Dice the chicken breast into small bits—about ¹/₂-inch (1.3 cm) cubes—and add it to the pot.

Take the shredding disc out of the food processor, put the S-blade in place, and put the celery, carrot, and onion, cut into a few big hunks, in the food processor bowl. Pulse to chop to a medium-fine consistency.

Melt the butter in a medium-size heavy skillet over medium-high heat and add the vegetables and the poultry seasoning. Sauté, stirring frequently.

When the microwave goes "ding," pull the cauliflower out of the microwave and add it to the soup. You can add the other veggies straight from the skillet or if you'd like them to be a little softer, put them in the bowl you cooked the cauliflower in, add a tablespoon (15 ml) of the broth from the soup, cover, and microwave them for 3 to 4 minutes on High before adding them to the soup.

Either way, stir the vegetables into the soup, salt and pepper to taste, and serve.

Yield: 3 or 4 servings. Assuming 3 servings, each will have 6 grams of carbohydrates and 1 gram of fiber, for a total of 5 grams of usable carbs and 28 grams of protein.

Note: If you'd prefer, you can make this with egg threads instead of the cauliflower rice, and it will be higher in protein. Just beat a couple of eggs in a measuring cup and pour the beaten egg over the simmering soup, stirring slowly with a fork.

⊕ Souper Easy, Souper Quick

How much simpler could this get? It's a great, warming starter for an otherwise very low carb meal.

 2 cups (475 ml) chicken broth

 2 teaspoons chopped garlic

 1 can (14 1/2 ounces, or 410 g) diced tomatoes

 2 tablespoons (28 g) jarred pesto

Put the chicken broth, garlic, and canned tomatoes, juice and all, in a 4 cup (950 ml) glass measuring cup. Microwave on high for 6 to 8 minutes or until good and hot. Pour into two bowls or four mugs and put a dollop of jarred pesto in each serving.

Yield: 2 to 4 servings, assuming 2, each will have 96 calories, 2 grams fat, 7 grams protein, 15 grams carbohydrate, trace dietary fiber, and 15 grams usable carb.

Note: This is endlessly variable. Add diced leftover chicken or turkey to make this into a main dish. Use beef broth and browned and crumbled ground beef for another version. Use tomatoes with green chilies, leave out the pesto, and add a handful of shredded Monterey Jack or 6 cheese Mexican blend for yet another version. Play around!

⏱ Chicken Noodle Soup with Sage Pesto

I adapted this from a recipe by Bobby Flay. I both speeded it up and slashed the carbs. Given the pedigree, it's not surprising it's really good!

1 quart (950 ml) chicken broth

1/2 cup (50 g) walnuts

1/2 cup (30 g) parsley sprigs

2 tablespoons (5 g) fresh sage

1/2 teaspoon chopped garlic

1/4 cup (60 ml) olive oil, divided

1/3 cup (33 g) grated Parmesan cheese

12 ounces (340 g) boneless, skinless chicken breast

2 teaspoons chicken bouillon concentrate

salt and pepper

1 packet tofu shirataki, fettuccini width

parsley

Pour your broth into a big saucepan and put it over high heat.

Spread your walnuts in a Pyrex pie plate and nuke them on high for 2 minutes.

While that's happening, assemble the parsley, sage, garlic, olive oil, and 1/4 cup (25 g) of the Parmesan in your food processor with the S-blade in place.

When the nuts are toasted, add them to the food processor and run until you have a paste.

Dice your chicken breast into 1/4 inch (6 cm) cubes—this is easier if it's partially frozen. Stir them into the broth, which should be getting hot by now. Stir in the bouillion concentrate, too, and salt and pepper to taste.

Drain your shirataki and rinse. Snip across them a couple of times with your kitchen shears and then add them to the soup.

When it's simmering and the chicken cubes are white through, serve. Add a couple of tablespoons (28 g) of the pesto to each bowl and top with the remaining cheese and parsley.

Yield: 3 servings, each with 525 calories, 38 grams fat, 41 grams protein, 6 grams carbohydrate, 1 gram dietary fiber, and 5 grams usable carb.

☺ Cheater's Chowder

This is so called because you're cheating on the usual ingredients, and you sure are cheating on the cooking time! You are not, however, cheating on your diet. This filling soup is a meal in itself.

> 1/4 head cauliflower
>
> 1 medium turnip (just bigger than a tennis ball)
>
> 3 slices bacon
>
> 1/2 medium onion
>
> 2 cups (475 ml) half-and-half
>
> 1 can (10 ounces, or 280 g) minced clams
>
> Salt or Vege-Sal and pepper

Whack the cauliflower into a few good-size chunks and put it in your food processor with the S-blade in place. Peel the turnip, quarter it, and drop it in, too. Pulse the processor until everything's chopped to a medium-fine consistency. Put the cauliflower and turnip in a microwaveable casserole with a lid, add a couple of tablespoons (28 ml) of water, cover, and microwave on High for 12 minutes.

While that's cooking, chop up the bacon (I snip mine up with cooking shears, right into the pot) and start frying it over medium-high heat in a large, heavy-bottomed saucepan, stirring from time to time.

Put that food processor bowl back on its base with the S-blade in place, throw in the half-onion, and pulse until the onion's chopped medium-fine. Dump the onion in with the bacon, which should be giving off some grease by now. Fry the onion and bacon together until the onion is translucent.

Pour the half-and-half and the clams into the pot—don't bother to drain the clams —stir it and then let the whole thing come to a simmer, stirring from time to time.

When the cauliflower and turnips are done, add them to the pot, too—no need to drain. Stir them in, salt and pepper it to taste, let the soup simmer just another minute or two, and serve.

Yield: 3 servings, each with 16 grams of carbohydrates and 1 gram of fiber, for a total of 15 grams of usable carbs and 31 grams of protein.

By the way, I tried running the nutritional analysis for this soup using half heavy cream in place of the half-and-half. It only cut 1 gram of carb off each serving— but it added 175 calories. Not worth it, if you ask me.

☉ Sopa Aguacate

With one of the quesadillas from chapter 2 on the side (see page 60), this makes a nice light supper.

    1 quart (950 ml) chicken broth
    1 ripe avocado
    2 scallions
    2 canned green chilies or 1 or 2 canned jalapeños, if you like it hot!
    2 tablespoons (2 g) chopped cilantro
    1/2 teaspoon salt or Vege-Sal

Start heating the broth—you can put it in a pan on the stove or you can put it in a large microwaveable container in the microwave.

While the broth is heating, scoop the avocado out of its skin and into a food processor with the S-blade in place. Add the scallions, peppers, cilantro, and salt. Pulse to chop everything together—you can leave a few chunks of avocado or purée it smooth, whichever you prefer.

When the broth is hot, divide the avocado mixture between 4 smallish soup bowls. Ladle the hot broth over the avocado mixture and serve.

Yield: 4 servings, each with 6 grams of carbohydrates and 3 grams of fiber, for a total of 3 grams of usable carbs and 6 grams of protein.

Bonus: You'll get a whopping 572 milligrams potassium and only 125 calories!

☉ Curried Chicken and Tomato Soup

This is just astonishingly good and even better considering how quick and easy it is. Next time you come home tired and hungry on a cold, rainy night, try this and discover true contentment.

>   3 cups (700 ml) chicken broth
>
>   1 can (14 1/2 ounces, or 410 g) diced tomatoes with green chilies
>
>   8 ounces (225 g) boneless, skinless chicken breast
>
>   1 tablespoon (14 g) butter
>
>   1 1/2 tablespoons (9 g) curry powder
>
>   1 can (13 1/2 ounces, or 395 g) coconut milk
>
>   1 teaspoon chicken bouillon concentrate
>
>   guar, xanthan, or glucomannan

In a large microwaveable dish or measuring cup, combine the chicken broth and canned tomatoes with chilies. Nuke on high for 5 minutes.

In the meantime, dice your chicken breast; you want cubes 1/4 to 1/2 inches (6 to 13 cm). Then, in a large saucepan, sauté the curry powder in the butter over low heat.

Pull out your chicken broth/tomato mixture, which should be hot by now, and pour it over the curry powder. Stir it up and turn up the burner to medium high. Stir in the coconut milk and the chicken bouillon concentrate. Thicken the whole thing up a little with your guar, xanthan, or glucomannan shaker; you want it a little thicker than heavy cream.

When your soup is getting to the simmering point, stir in the diced chicken. Don't just plunk it in and let it sit or it'll congeal in a lump in the bottom of the pot. Stir it in so each cube cooks separately.

It shouldn't take more than a minute or two for those little bitty chicken cubes to be cooked. Serve it up!

Yield: 3 servings, each with 366 calories, 29 grams fat, 20 grams protein, 11 grams carbohydrate, 3 grams dietary fiber, and 8 grams usable carb.

chapter twelve

15~Minute Condiments, Sauces, Dressings, and Seasonings

When you read the labels, you'll be stunned at how much sugar you'll find in condiments, sauces, salad dressings, and even some sprinkle-on seasonings. Fortunately, it's quite quick and simple to make your own.

Many of these condiments, sauces, dressings, and seasonings are called for in other recipes in the book. Others are not but are included because they offer great, easy ways to season the simple slabs of protein—chicken breasts, fish fillets, steaks, chops, and so on—that are the staples of quick low-carb cooking.

You'll find some new recipes here, plus a few I've repeated from *500 Low-Carb Recipes*—the ones I thought would be most helpful for making quick and varied meals.

Dipping Sauces

Dipping sauces are an increasingly popular way to add variety to simple foods—even McDonald's offers dipping sauces with their McNuggets! Each of these dipping sauces is called for in another recipe in this book, but feel free to use them any way you like.

☺ "Honey" Mustard Dipping Sauce

Great with the fried *Chicken Tenders* (see page 90) or with a simple chicken breast or pork chop.

> 1/4 cup (60 g) mayonnaise
>
> 2 tablespoons (22 g) spicy mustard
>
> 1 teaspoon Splenda

Simply combine everything and you're all set.

Yield: Makes a little more than 1/3 cup (about 85 g), or enough for about 4 people eating *Chicken Tenders*. Each serving has 1 gram of carbohydrates, no fiber, and 1 gram of protein.

☺ Apricot Ginger Dipping Sauce

Also great with *Chicken Tenders* (see page 90)—or anything else you might use the "Honey" Mustard Dipping Sauce on—only it tastes a lot different.

> 1/4 cup (60 g) mayonnaise
>
> 1 1/2 tablespoons (30 g) low-sugar apricot preserves
>
> 1 teaspoon grated gingerroot
>
> 1/4 teaspoon minced garlic or 1/2 clove garlic, crushed
>
> 1/2 teaspoon Splenda
>
> 3/4 teaspoon soy sauce

Simply combine everything.

Yield: Makes just under 1/3 cup (about 85 g), or enough for about 4 people eating *Chicken Tenders*. Each serving has 3 grams of carbohydrates, with a trace of fiber and protein.

⊕ Asian Dipping Sauce

This is perfect with the *Lettuce Wraps* on page 101, but it's also good with *Chicken Tenders* (see page 90), or whatever you have on hand.

1/4 cup (6 g) Splenda

1/4 cup (60 ml) water

2 tablespoons (28 ml) soy sauce

2 tablespoons (28 ml) rice vinegar

2 tablespoons (30 g) Dana's No-Sugar Ketchup (see page 309)
   or commercial sugar-free ketchup

1 tablespoon (15 ml) lemon juice

1/4 teaspoon toasted sesame oil

2 teaspoons dry mustard

2 teaspoons chili garlic paste

Just assemble everything in a blender and run it until everything's well combined. If you don't use it all up at once, keep in a tightly sealed container in the fridge and it will last a week, at least.

Yield: Makes roughly 3/4 cup (170 ml), or 6 servings of 2 tablespoons (28 g) each. Each serving has 3 grams of carbohydrates, a trace of fiber, and 1 gram of protein.

⊕ Nuoc Cham

This sweet-tart-spicy dipping sauce is purely Vietnamese and absolutely wonderful! It's essential for the *Lemon Chicken* (see page 83) and the Vietnamese *Chicken Salad* (see page 173), but once you try this, you'll think of all sorts of ways to use it.

> 2 tablespoons (36 g) fish sauce
>
> 2 tablespoons (28 ml) lime juice
>
> 1 1/2 teaspoons rice vinegar
>
> 3 tablespoons (4.5 g) Splenda
>
> 1/2 teaspoon minced garlic or 1 clove garlic, crushed
>
> 1 teaspoon chili garlic paste

Simply combine everything in a small dish.

Yield: About 1/3 cup (85 g), or 4 or 5 servings. Assuming 4 servings, each will have 4 grams of carbohydrates, a trace of fiber, and a trace of protein. (And approximately 15 metric boatloads of flavor!)

⊕ Stir-Fry Sauce

If you like Chinese food, make this up and keep it on hand. Then you can just throw any sort of meat and vegetables in your wok or skillet and have a meal in minutes.

> 1/2 cup (120 ml) soy sauce
>
> 1/2 cup (120 ml) dry sherry
>
> 2 cloves garlic, crushed, or 1 teaspoon minced garlic
>
> 2 tablespoons (16 g) grated fresh ginger
>
> 2 teaspoons Splenda

Simply combine everything and store in a tightly sealed container in the refrigerator.

Yield: Makes 1 cup (225 g). Use about 1 1/2 to 2 tablespoons (23 to 28 g) per serving of stir-fry. Each serving contains 2 grams of carbohydrates, no fiber, and no protein.

⊕ Easy Remoulade Sauce

This is good on anything fishy or seafoodlike.

> 1 cup (225 g) mayonnaise
>
> 2 tablespoons (22 g) spicy brown or Dijon mustard
>
> 2 tablespoons (28 ml) lemon juice
>
> 1 teaspoon dried tarragon, crumbled
>
> 2 tablespoons (18 g) capers, drained and chopped a bit

Just stir everything up, and you're good to go!

Yield: Makes about 1 1/3 cups (310 g), or 5 servings of just under 1/4 cup (55 g) each. Each serving has 1 gram of carbohydrates, a trace of fiber, and 1 gram of protein.

⊕ Lemon-Basil Cream Sauce

This dish is so summery!

> 2 tablespoons (28 g) butter
>
> 1 teaspoon chopped garlic
>
> 4 ounces (115 g) cream cheese
>
> 1 cup (235 ml) heavy cream
>
> 1 lemon
>
> 2 tablespoons (5 g) minced fresh basil
>
> salt and pepper

Put a saucepan over lowest heat. Melt the butter and start the garlic sautéing in it—be careful it doesn't brown at all. Just sauté it a couple of minutes over very low heat.

Cut the cream cheese into small chunks and add it to the pan along with the heavy cream. You can goose the heat up a tiny bit, but keep it quite low. Scorching is a big no-no.

While the cream warms and the cheese melts, grate a teaspoon of zest from your lemon and mince your basil.

Go stir your sauce! When the cheese is melted and it's all smooth, add the lemon zest and squeeze in the juice of the lemon. Now stir in the basil.

Salt and pepper to taste and serve over tofu shirataki fettuccini, chicken breast, shrimp, sole—you name it.

Yield: 4 servings, each with 361 calories, 38 grams fat, 4 grams protein, 5 grams carbohydrate, trace dietary fiber, and 5 grams usable carb.

⊕ Salsa Nortena

This is my clone of a sauce I bought on a trip to Mexico. It's great on omelets, chicken, or pork chops and steaks.

8 fluid ounces (235 ml) tomato sauce

1/2 cup (130 g) natural peanut butter

1/2 teaspoon chopped garlic

1 teaspoon ground cumin

2 chipotle chiles canned in adobo

1/2 cup (120 ml) chicken broth or 1/2 cup (120 ml) water and 1/2 teaspoon chicken bouillon concentrate

salt to taste

Just assemble everything in your food processor or blender and run until it's smooth, scraping down the sides as needed. Store in a snap-top container in the fridge.

Yield: 8 servings, each with 106 calories, 8 grams fat, 4 grams protein, 6 grams carbohydrate, 2 grams dietary fiber, and 4 grams usable carb.

Butter

⊕Mustard-Shallot Butter

This is great on steaks, burgers, chicken, or fish.

2 shallots

2 tablespoons (22 g) spicy brown or Dijon mustard

1 teaspoon lemon juice

1/2 cup (112 g) butter, softened

1/4 teaspoon salt (optional)

Put the shallots in your food processor with the S-blade in place and run until they're finely chopped. Add everything else and run until it's all well-mixed. The classical way to serve something like this is to chill it in a roll and then slice it. But for a fifteen minute meal, who's got that kind of time? Just scoop it into a little dish and let everyone spoon a dollop or two over their steak or burger.

Yield: 4 servings, each with 214 calories, 24 grams fat, 1 gram protein, 1 gram carbohydrate, trace dietary fiber, and 1 gram usable carb.

⊕ Bacon Butter

Take that, Dean Ornish! This is great on steaks or burgers, but try it melted over fried eggs, too.

> 4 slices bacon
>
> 1/2 cup (112 g) butter
>
> 1 teaspoon spicy brown or Dijon mustard

Lay your bacon on a microwave bacon rack or in a glass pie plate. Microwave on high for 4 to 5 minutes or until crisp.

In the meantime, throw your butter in your food processor and add the mustard. Pulse until well combined.

By now your bacon is done. Pull it out of the microwave and use your kitchen shears to snip it into the food processor in little bits. Pulse the food processor to mix in the bacon. The more you pulse, the finer the bacon bits will be; go by your own taste.

Yield: 4 servings, each with 120 calories, 13 grams fat, 1 gram protein, trace carbohydrate, trace dietary fiber, and virtually no usable carbs.

Salad Dressings

When you're pressed for time or just avoiding cooking, you're likely to use bottled salad dressing. No reason not to, so long as you stick to the low-carb varieties. However, I'm including two salad dressing recipes, the first because it's so unusual and it's used in a few recipes elsewhere in this book, and the second—a repeat from *500 Low-Carb Recipes*—because coleslaw is tremendously popular, yet so often sugary.

☺ Guacamole Dressing

This is guacamole thinned out just enough to make a salad dressing—wonderful! Remember, the little black avocados are much lower in carbs than the big green ones. Do use this dressing up pretty quickly; you know how avocado changes color. If you must keep the leftovers for a day, store them in a tightly sealed container in the refrigerator.

> 1 ripe avocado
>
> 1/2 cup (115 g) plain yogurt
>
> 1/4 cup (60 ml) olive oil
>
> 1 tablespoon (15 ml) lime juice
>
> 1/2 teaspoon minced garlic or 1 clove garlic, crushed
>
> 1/4 teaspoon hot sauce
>
> 1/4 teaspoon salt

Cut the avocado in half, remove the seed, and scoop the flesh into a blender or food processor. Add the yogurt, olive oil, lime juice, garlic, hot sauce, and salt and blend until smooth.

Yield: 4 servings, each with 6 grams of carbohydrates and 2 grams of fiber, for a total of 4 grams of usable carbs (actually less if you use the *GO-Diet's* figure of 4 grams of carbohydrates per cup [225 ml] of plain yogurt) and 3 grams of protein.

✷ A serving of this dressing packs more potassium than a banana!

⊕ Coleslaw Dressing

Virtually all commercial coleslaw dressing is simply full of sugar, which is a shame, since cabbage is a very low-carb vegetable. I just love coleslaw, so I had to come up with a sugar-free dressing! Make this up, pour it over a bag or two of pre-shredded coleslaw mix, and you'll have a great, versatile side dish in no time. Always try to make lots of coleslaw; it gets better over the day or two after it's made.

> ¹/₂ cup (115 g) mayonnaise
>
> ¹/₂ cup (115 g) sour cream
>
> 1 to 1 ¹/₂ tablespoons (15 to 23 ml) apple cider vinegar
>
> 1 to 1 ¹/₂ teaspoons prepared mustard
>
> ¹/₂ to 1 teaspoon salt or Vege-Sal
>
> ¹/₂ to 1 packet artificial sweetener, or Splenda

Just mix it all together, and you're all set!

Yield: Assuming that you get 12 servings out of a batch, this dressing will add only 1 gram of carbohydrates to each serving, plus a trace of fiber and protein.

Variation: You may, of course, vary these proportions to taste. Also, a teaspoon or so of celery seed can be nice in this. This much would be enough for at least two bags of coleslaw mix, as far as I'm concerned, but use an amount to suit your taste.

☉ Cajun Dressing

This quantity is right for the *Cajun Chicken Salad* (see page 174), but feel free to quadruple it and keep it in the fridge. It would be good on a wedge of iceberg lettuce, for dipping shrimp in, or any manner of things.

> ¹/₄ cup (60 g) mayonnaise
>
> 1 teaspoon sugar-free ketchup (Make your own from the recipe on page 309 or purchase, whichever you like.)
>
> 1 sugar-free bread and butter pickle slice
>
> 1 teaspoon Cajun seasoning
>
> ¹/₄ teaspoon onion powder
>
> ¹/₄ teaspoon chopped garlic
>
> 1 dash Worcestershire sauce
>
> 1 dash Tabasco sauce or other Louisiana-style hot sauce

Just run everything through the food processor until the pickle's chopped up. That's it!

Yield: 3 servings, each with 138 calories, 16 grams fat, trace protein, 2 grams carbohydrate, trace dietary fiber, and 2 grams usable carb.

☺ Maple-Bacon Vinaigrette

Oh, man, is this good. Start saving your bacon grease! This is great on any salad. It is especially good with the *Spinach Salad with Maple Glazed Bacon, Nectarines, and Feta* (see page 257).

2 tablespoons (28 ml) olive oil

2 tablespoons (28 g) bacon grease

2 tablespoons (28 ml) cider vinegar

2 teaspoons spicy brown or Dijon mustard

1/2 shallot

2 teaspoons sugar-free pancake syrup

1/4 teaspoon chopped garlic

1/4 teaspoon salt

Simply assemble everything in your blender or food processor and run until it's creamy. Pour it over your salad and toss.

Yield: 3 to 4 servings, assuming 3, each will have 166 calories, 18 grams fat, trace protein, 1 gram carbohydrate, trace dietary fiber, 1 gram usable carb.

Sprinkle-On Seasonings

Sprinkle-on seasonings are a simple way to vary "chicken again, chops again, steak again" and the like. There are many good varieties to choose from in your grocery store, and I urge you to put together a modest collection! However, if you'd like to make your own, they're very little work for a lot of result—plus, when you make sprinkle-on seasonings yourself, you know that they're sugar-free. Here are some I've come up with that I like.

☻ Many-Pepper Steak Seasoning

This adds real zing to a steak without covering up the flavor. Make this up, keep it in a shaker, and you'll be ready to cook a really special steak at a moment's notice.

>   1 tablespoon (7 g) onion powder
>
>   3 tablespoons (27 g) garlic powder
>
>   3 tablespoons (21 g) paprika
>
>   1 tablespoon (3 g) oregano
>
>   1 1/2 tablespoons (9 g) pepper
>
>   2 teaspoons lemon pepper
>
>   1 teaspoon cayenne—or more if you like it really hot!

Simply combine everything well and put it in a shaker. Sprinkle liberally over both sides of a steak before broiling or grilling.

Yield: This is enough to season 12 to 15 steaks. Assuming 15 steaks, each will have 3 grams of carbohydrates and 1 gram of fiber, or for a total of 2 grams of carbs to a whole steak—and that steak is likely to be 2 or more servings, so figure 1 gram per serving—and no fiber or protein.

⊕ Dana's Chicken Seasoning

This is wonderful sprinkled over a chicken breast before grilling or as a table seasoning for any poultry. (It's also great sprinkled over whole or cut-up chicken before roasting, but that doesn't fit into our 15-minute time frame.)

3 tablespoons (54 g) salt

1 teaspoon paprika

1 teaspoon onion powder

1 teaspoon garlic powder

1 teaspoon curry powder

1/2 teaspoon black pepper

Combine all the ingredients thoroughly and store in a salt shaker or the shaker from an old container of herbs. Simply sprinkle over chicken before roasting; I use it to season at the table, as well.

Yield: Makes just over 1/4 cup (55 g). In the whole recipe, there are only 7 grams of carbohydrates and 1 gram of fiber, for a total of 6 grams of usable carbs and no protein—so the amount of carbohydrates in the teaspoon or so you sprinkle over a piece of chicken is negligible.

⊕ Cajun Seasoning

This sprinkle-on seasoning will liven up chops, steaks, chicken, fish—just about anything!

> 2 1/2 tablespoons (18 g) paprika
>
> 2 tablespoons (36 g) salt
>
> 2 tablespoons (18 g) garlic powder
>
> 1 tablespoon (6 g) black pepper
>
> 1 tablespoon (7 g) onion powder
>
> 1 tablespoon (5 g) cayenne pepper
>
> 1 tablespoon (3 g) dried oregano
>
> 1 tablespoon (3 g) dried thyme

Combine all the ingredients thoroughly and keep in an air-tight container.

Yield: Makes 2/3 cup (90 g). In this whole recipe, there are 37 grams of carbohydrates and 9 grams of fiber, for a total of 28 grams of usable carbs and no protein. Considering how spicy this is, you're unlikely to use more than a teaspoon or two at a time. One teaspoon has 1 gram of carbohydrates, a trace of fiber, and no protein.

⊕Jerk Seasoning

Sprinkle this over chicken, pork chops, or fish before cooking for an instant hit of hot, sweet, spicy flavor.

> 1 tablespoon (5 g) onion flakes
>
> 2 teaspoons ground thyme
>
> 1 teaspoon ground allspice
>
> 1/4 teaspoon ground cinnamon
>
> 1 teaspoon black pepper
>
> 1 teaspoon cayenne pepper
>
> 1 tablespoon (7 g) onion powder
>
> 2 teaspoons salt
>
> 1/4 teaspoon ground nutmeg
>
> 2 tablespoons (3 g) Splenda

Combine all the ingredients and store in an air-tight container.

Yield: Makes about 1/3 cup (30 g). If you use 1 teaspoon, it will have 1 gram of carbohydrates, a trace of fiber, and no protein.

☉ Wonderful Memphis-Style Dry Rub BBQ

A *Lowcarbezine!* reader who didn't supply his or her name sent this recipe, so we refer to them simply as the Mystery Chef. This is great on ribs, chops, or chicken and far lower-carb than barbecue sauce.

> 1 tablespoon (7 g) paprika
>
> 2 teaspoons chili powder
>
> 3/4 teaspoon salt
>
> 1/4 teaspoon dry mustard
>
> 1/4 teaspoon garlic powder
>
> 1/8 teaspoon pepper

Mix all the ingredients together and store in a salt shaker. Sprinkle on both sides of whatever meat you're cooking, and grill.

Yield: This makes enough for 3 1/2 pounds (1.6 kg) of ribs, or about 3 servings. If, indeed, 3 of you eat all of this recipe, each will get 2 grams of carbohydrates and 1 gram of fiber, for a total of 1 gram of usable carbs, no fiber, and no protein. By contrast, your average commercial barbecue sauce has between 10 and 15 grams per 2-tablespoon (32 g) serving—and who ever stopped at 2 tablespoons (32 g)?

☉ Southwestern Steak Rub

> 1 tablespoon (8 g) chili powder
>
> 1 teaspoon garlic powder
>
> 1 teaspoon onion powder
>
> 1/2 teaspoon oregano
>
> 1/4 teaspoon Splenda

Just mix everything together and sprinkle liberally on both sides of a steak before pan-broiling. This is enough for a couple of good-sized steaks. It would be good for seasoning burgers, too.

Yield: The whole batch contains 43 calories, 1 gram fat, 2 grams protein, 8 grams carbohydrate, 3 grams dietary fiber, and 5 grams usable fiber.

☺ Chili-Cocoa Rub

I was originally going to use this recipe in the context of Chili-Cocoa Rubbed Steak. Then I tried this rub on pork and chicken and realized it was way too good to limit that way. Make this up, keep it in a shaker by the stove, and use it to improve all manner of things! It's the best rub I've come up with in a long time.

> 1/4 cup (72 g) salt or Vege-Sal
>
> 2 tablespoons (3 g) Splenda granular
>
> 1 tablespoon (15 g) erythritol
>
> 2 teaspoons cocoa powder
>
> 3 tablespoons (27 g) garlic powder
>
> 1 tablespoon (7 g) onion powder
>
> 3 tablespoons (21 g) cumin
>
> 2 tablespoons (23 g) chili powder
>
> 2 tablespoons (12 g) pepper

Stir everything together and store in a used spice-shaker bottle. Use on steaks, pork chops, burgers, ribs—you name it. It's so good!

Yield: Figure this for 16 servings, each with 17 calories, trace fat (20.9% calories from fat), 1 gram protein, 3 grams carbohydrate, 1 gram dietary fiber, and 2 grams usable carb.

Condiments

Did you know that ketchup has more sugar than ice cream does? You can buy no-sugar ketchup, but it's pricey—and it's not worth it when making your own is such a snap. And once you've got ketchup in the fridge, you can make steak sauce and cocktail sauce. Clearly it is in your best interests to put together a batch of ketchup today!

Commercial barbecue sauce is, I'm sorry to say, even more syrupy than ketchup; so much so that it's very hard to fit most commercial barbecue sauces into your diet. You'll find a recipe for barbecue sauce below, but it's a bit more trouble than the ketchup. There are a few low- or no-sugar barbecue sauces on the market. My favorite is Stubb's, out of Austin, Texas, which has about half the sugar of most commercial barbecue sauces yet tastes at least as good, if not better. It's worth checking your grocery store condiment aisle for it. Walden's is a brand marketed directly to the low-carb market; low-carb e-tailers (online retailers) carry this. I like Stubb's better, but Walden's is lower carb. Atkins also makes a barbecue sauce, but I haven't tried it yet.

☺ Dana's No-Sugar Ketchup

This great-tasting ketchup has all the flavor of your favorite brand, without the high carb count. The guar or xanthan isn't essential, but it makes your ketchup a little thicker and helps keep the water from separating out if you don't use it up quickly.

1 can (6 ounces, or 170 g) can tomato paste

2/3 cup (160 ml) cider vinegar

1/3 cup (80 ml) water

1/3 cup (8 g) Splenda

2 tablespoons (20 g) finely minced onion

2 cloves garlic, crushed

1 teaspoon salt or Vege-Sal

1/8 teaspoon ground allspice

1/8 teaspoon ground cloves

1/8 teaspoon pepper

1/4 teaspoon guar or xanthan

Assemble everything in a blender and run the blender—you'll have to scrape down the sides because this mixture is thick—until the bits of onion disappear. Store in a tightly sealed container in the refrigerator.

Yield: Makes 1 1/2 cups (360 g) of ketchup, or twenty-four 1-tablespoon (15 g) servings. Each serving will have 2.25 grams of carbohydrates, a trace of fiber, and a trace of protein.

⊕ Low-Carb Steak Sauce

If you have *Dana's No-Sugar Ketchup* on hand, this is a cinch to make. It's nice to have on hand if you're having a simple broiled steak, and it's indispensable with steak and eggs.

> ¼ cup (60 g) Dana's No-Sugar Ketchup *see previous page*
>
> 1 tablespoon (15 ml) Worcestershire sauce
>
> 1 teaspoon lemon juice

Simply combine the ingredients well. Store in a tightly sealed container in the refrigerator.

Yield: Makes five 1 tablespoon (15 g) servings, each with 2.25 grams of carbohydrates, a trace of fiber, and a trace of protein.

⊕ Cocktail Sauce

If you like shrimp, frozen, cooked, peeled shrimp are a terrific convenience food—but it's nice to have something to dip them in. Commercial cocktail sauce, like so many other condiments, is full of sugar; you'll save quite a few carbs by making your own.

> ¼ cup (60 g) *Dana's No-Sugar Ketchup see previous page*
>
> 1 teaspoon prepared horseradish

Just stir together and dip!

Yield: The whole batch has about 9 grams of carbohydrates, a trace of fiber, and no protein.

> **Note:** Mustard and mayonnaise, mixed together, also make a nice dip for shrimp. Or you could buy Dijonnaise. Either way, this mustard-mayo combo is lower in carbs than even the sugar-free cocktail sauce. Try dipping shrimp in *Nuoc Cham* (see page 292), too.

⊕ Reduced-Carb Spicy Barbecue Sauce

Ketchup is bad enough, but barbecue sauce has even more sugar! Make your own. This is, I confess, the only recipe in the book that takes more than 15 minutes—the idea is to have it hanging around in the refrigerator, ready to call on for making Slow Cooker "Barbecued" Ribs (see page 226) and the like. However, if you can find Walden's, Stubb's, or any other reasonably low-carb commercial barbecue sauce, I'll understand if you ignore this recipe.

1 clove garlic, crushed

1 small onion, finely minced

4 tablespoons (55 g) butter or oil

4 tablespoons (6 g) Splenda

2 teaspoons blackstrap molasses

1 teaspoon salt or Vege-Sal

1 teaspoon dry mustard

1 teaspoon paprika

1 teaspoon chili powder

1/2 teaspoon black pepper

1 1/2 cups (355 ml) water

1/4 cup (60 ml) cider vinegar

1 tablespoon (15 ml) Worcestershire sauce

1 tablespoon (15 g) prepared horseradish

1 tablespoon (15 ml) liquid smoke*

1 can (6 ounces, or 170g) tomato paste

* Most big grocery stores carry this. A company called Colgin makes it.

In a saucepan, cook the onion and garlic in the butter or oil for a few minutes. Stir in the Splenda, molasses, salt, dry mustard, paprika, chili powder, black pepper, water, vinegar, Worcestershire sauce, and horseradish. Let it simmer for 15 to 20 minutes. Then whisk in the tomato paste and smoke flavoring, and let it simmer for another 5 to 10 minutes. Store in a jar in the refrigerator.

Yield: This makes about 2 2/3 cups (625 g) of sauce, or about twenty-one 2-tablespoon (32 g) servings, each with 3 grams of carbohydrates and 1 gram of fiber, for a total of 2 grams of usable carbs, no fiber, and no protein.

Marinades

Marinating things, simple though it may be, actually takes us well beyond our 15-minute time limit. So why include these two recipes from *500 Low-Carb Recipes*? Because both of them are good when used in our quick cooking, too. Brushing a little *Tequila Lime Marinade* over a chicken breast before sautéing it and then spooning a little more over it as it cooks adds a lot of flavor. You could also use the *Tequila Lime Marinade* to flavor sautéed shrimp. As for the *Teriyaki Marinade*, why not use it with some ribs, chicken, or pork loin in your slow cooker? You'll find a recipe in the slow cooker section where you do exactly that.

⊙Tequila Lime Marinade

This is great for boneless, skinless chicken breasts, fish, and shrimp. If you don't have time to marinade, you could pour a little into a skillet while sautéing.

> 1/3 cup (80 ml) lime juice, bottled or fresh
>
> 1/3 cup (80 ml) water
>
> 3 tablespoon (45 ml) tequila
>
> 1 tablespoon (1.5 g) Splenda
>
> 1 tablespoon (15 ml) soy sauce
>
> 2 cloves garlic, crushed

Combine all of the ingredients and refrigerate until use.

Yield: This makes roughly 3/4 cup (175 ml)—enough for a dozen boneless, skinless chicken breasts or a couple of pounds (900 g) of shrimp. The whole batch has 13 grams of carbohydrates and 1 gram of fiber, for a total of 12 grams of usable carbs, no fiber, and no protein. But since you drain most of the marinade off, you won't actually get more than a gram or two of carbs.

⊕Teriyaki Sauce

This is good on chicken, beef, fish—just about anything!

1/2 cup (120 ml) soy sauce

1/4 cup (60 ml) dry sherry

1 clove garlic, crushed

2 tablespoons (3 g) Splenda

1 tablespoon (8 g) grated fresh ginger

Simply combine all of the ingredients and refrigerate until use.

Yield: Makes just over 3/4 cup (175 ml), or almost twelve 1-tablespoon (15 ml) servings, each with about 3 grams of carbohydrates, no fiber, and no protein.

⊕ Apple Walnut Dressing

This dressing has no grain of any kind in it and still tastes great. Serve with a simple poultry or pork dish.

4 tablespoons (55 g) butter

1 crisp, tart apple (I use a Granny Smith because I like the flavor,
   but one with a red skin would look prettier.)

2 large stalks celery

1 medium onion

1 cup (100 g) shelled walnuts

8 ounces (225 g) sliced mushrooms

3/4 teaspoon salt or Vege-Sal

1 1/2 teaspoons poultry seasoning

Melt the butter in a large, heavy skillet over medium heat.

Quarter the apple and trim out the core, whack each quarter in half (making eighths), and drop them in your food processor with the S-blade in place. Whack each stalk of celery into 4 or 5 big chunks and throw them in, too. Quarter the onion, peel it, and throw it in and then dump in the walnuts. Pulse the food processor until everything's a medium consistency.

Dump this mixture, along with the mushrooms (which we're assuming you bought already sliced—if not, just chop 'em with everything else), into the butter in the skillet, turn the heat up to medium-high, and sauté everything for a minute or two, stirring. Then cover it and let it cook for 10 minutes, uncovering every 3 minutes or so to stir the whole thing again.

Stir in the salt and poultry seasoning, let it cook for another minute or two, and serve.

Yield: 6 to 8 servings. Assuming 6 servings, each will have 9 grams of carbohydrates and 3 grams of fiber, for a total of 6 grams of usable carbs and 6 grams of protein.

15~Minute Beverages

Coffee Drinks

If you're fond of coffee, try laying in a supply of either flavored coffees (the kind you actually brew, *not* the General Mills International Coffees, which contain sugar and other objectionable ingredients) and sugar-free coffee flavoring syrups (Da Vinci Sugar Free is probably the most widely available; look at your local gourmet coffee take-out joint, but Torani and Monin O'Free are also fine). Combine these with some heavy cream, if you like, to make an endless array of coffee drinks. Use decaf if you find that caffeine after dinner keeps you awake.

Here are some ideas to jump-start your coffee creativity

⊕ Irish Coffee

I included this in *500 Low-Carb Recipes*, but it seemed too classic to omit here.

> 1 shot (1 ½ ounces, 45 ml) Irish whiskey*
>
> 6 ounces hot coffee (170 ml)
>
> Splenda to taste
>
> Whipped cream (See *Whipped Topping* recipe, page 31)

* You may as well use cheap, blended whiskey for this; use Jamieson's or Bushmill's, and you'll make my husband cry.

The traditional glass for this is a stemmed Irish coffee mug, but I wouldn't bother running out and buying them unless you're exceedingly fond of Irish coffee. Just put the shot of whiskey in a large mug, pour the coffee over it, add Splenda to taste, and top with a good dollop of whipped cream.

Yield: 1 serving. If you use 2 teaspoons of Splenda and a couple of tablespoons (28 g) of whipped cream, you'll get just 2 grams of carbohydrates, no fiber, and no protein.

⊕ Whipped Topping

This seems as good a place as any to repeat my favorite recipe for making whipped cream—the instant pudding in this recipe gives it a lovely, mild sweetness and a glorious texture. By the way, don't try to whip cream in your blender or food processor—it won't work. Use an electric mixer, an egg beater, or that old standby, the whisk. I think an electric mixer is best. Use this in coffee drinks, over berries, or anywhere else you think a little whipped cream might be nice. This recipe makes a lot; feel free to halve it.

> 1 cup (235 ml) heavy whipping cream, well chilled
> 1 tablespoon (15 g) sugar-free vanilla instant pudding powder

Simply whip the two together until you have fluffy, gorgeous whipped cream. Don't overbeat, or you'll get sweet vanilla butter.

Yield: This is enough for a crowd—2 cups (455 g), or 16 servings of 2 tablespoons (28 g), each with only a trace of carbohydrates, no fiber, and no protein.

Note: See the words "well chilled" after the cream in this recipe? That's because warm cream may well refuse to whip on you. Furthermore, your bowl and beaters shouldn't be warm, either. If they're fresh out of the dishwasher, chill them in the freezer for 5 to 10 minutes or at the very least run cold water over them and then dry them before making your *Whipped Topping*.

☉ Café Chantilly

This is a classic!

>1 tablespoon (15 ml) cognac
>
>4 ounces (120 ml) brewed coffee
>
>Unsweetened whipped cream (just whip chilled heavy cream by itself with an electric mixer)

Just stir the cognac into the coffee, top with a dollop of whipped cream, and serve.

Yield: 1 serving, with just 1 gram of carbohydrates, no fiber, and no protein.

✫ Each serving has only 65 calories!

☉ Mexican Coffee

Traditionally, this is made with pilloncillo sugar—Mexican brown sugar—and milk, but that's too many carbs for us. Here's the reduced-carb version.

>6 ounces (170 ml) brewed coffee
>
>2 to 3 tablespoons (28 to 45 ml) heavy cream
>
>2 teaspoons Splenda
>
>2 drops blackstrap molasses*
>
>Tiny pinch ground cinnamon
>
>Tiny pinch ground cloves

* It helps to keep your blackstrap in a squeeze bottle. I buy my blackstrap in bulk from my health food store and keep it in one of those "honey bears."

Pour the coffee and stir in the cream, Splenda, and molasses. Sprinkle the spices over the top and serve.

Yield: 1 serving, with 3 grams of carbohydrates, the merest trace of fiber, and 1 gram of protein.

⊕ Café Vienna

This is coffee for chocolate lovers or chocolate for coffee lovers.

> 6 ounces (170 ml) brewed coffee
>
> 2 tablespoons (30 g) sugar-free chocolate coffee flavoring syrup
>
> 2 tablespoons (28 ml) heavy cream
>
> Tiny pinch ground cinnamon

Pour the coffee, stir in the chocolate syrup and heavy cream, dust the cinnamon over the top, and serve.

Yield: 1 serving. Assuming you use Torani, Monin, or Da Vinci coffee flavoring syrup (which are made with Splenda instead of polyols), this will have 2 grams of carbohydrates, a trace of fiber, and 1 gram of protein.

Note: If you'd like to spiff this up for company, used whipped cream (see *Whipped Topping* on page 316) instead of the plain heavy cream.

⊕ Chocolate Orange Coffee

I came up with this one morning when my husband was out of cream for his coffee—it kept me from having to run out to the store before breakfast, and he loved it!

> 6 ounces (170 ml) brewed coffee
>
> 1 tablespoon (15 g) sugar-free chocolate coffee flavoring syrup
>
> 1 or 2 drops orange extract

Pour the coffee and stir in the syrup and the extract. That's all!

Yield: 1 serving. Again assuming you use Torani, Monin, or Da Vinci brand syrup, you'll have just 1 gram of carbohydrates here, no fiber, and no protein.

Café Incontro

This is for adults only, of course!

> 6 ounces (170 ml) brewed coffee
>
> 1 scant shot (1 ounce, or 28 ml) dark rum
>
> 2 teaspoons sugar-free chocolate coffee flavoring syrup
>
> Splenda to taste, if desired

Pour the coffee, add the rum, syrup, and Splenda, and serve. That's all!

Yield: 1 serving, with just 1 gram of carbohydrates (again, we're talking the Torani, Monin, or Da Vinci syrup), no fiber, and no protein. Add 0.5 grams of carbohydrates for each teaspoon of Splenda you add.

Sodas or Floats

These are American classics and are really quick and simple to make. You may, of course, use any flavor of no-sugar-added ice cream and any flavor of diet soda to make floats. These are just a few popular combinations. You can also use one of the sugar-free coffee-flavoring syrups plus seltzer or club soda in place of the diet soda, if you'd like to get really creative.

⊕ Root Beer Float

My sister keeps IBC Sugar-Free Root Beer and Dreyer's Vanilla No-Sugar-Added Ice Cream in the house for this purpose and this purpose alone.

> 1 small scoop vanilla no-sugar-added ice cream, vanilla flavor
>
> 1 can or bottle sugar-free root beer, well chilled

Put the ice cream in a large glass or mug and pour the root beer over it. Serve with straws and a long-handled spoon.

Yield: 1 serving; the carb count will depend on your brand of no-sugar-added ice cream.

⊕ Chocolate Float

If you can get chocolate-flavored diet soda in your region, this is a nice variant of the Root Beer Float.

>1 small scoop vanilla no-sugar-added ice cream, vanilla flavor
>
>1 can sugar-free chocolate-fudge flavored soda, well chilled

Put the ice cream in a large glass or mug and pour the soda over it. Serve with a straw and a long-handled spoon.

Yield: 1 serving; the carb count will depend on your brand of no-sugar-added ice cream.

Note: Canfield's makes diet chocolate-fudge flavored soda. If you can't find it in a local grocery store, there are several Websites that sell it. Be aware, however, that this is one of those love-it-or-hate-it products. Faygo also makes a chocolate soda.

⊕ Dreamsicle Float

If you were a fan of Dreamsicles as a kid, you'll love this float!

>1 small scoop no-sugar-added ice cream, vanilla flavor
>
>1 can sugar-free orange soda, well chilled

Put the ice cream in a large glass or mug and pour the soda over it. Serve with a straw and a long-handled spoon.

Yield: 1 serving; the carb count will depend on your brand of no-sugar-added ice cream.

⊕ Farmer's Soda

This is simpler than a float and a bit lower carb.

> 1/4 cup (60 ml) heavy cream
>
> 1 can sugar-free soda, flavor of your choice, well chilled

Simply pour the cream into the bottom of a large glass and pour the soda over it.

Yield: 1 serving, with 3 grams of carbohydrates, no fiber, and no protein.

⊕ Chocolate Ice Cream Soda

This is a true old-fashioned treat. Grab your sweetheart and two straws.

> 2 tablespoons (30 g) sugar-free chocolate coffee flavoring syrup
>
> 2 tablespoons (30 g) sugar-free Hershey's syrup
>
> 1/2 cup (70 g) sugar-free vanilla ice cream (I used Breyer's CarbSmart.)
>
> 6 fluid ounces (175 ml) club soda, chilled

Put the syrups in the bottom of a glass. Add the ice cream and pour the club soda over all. Use a straw if you have one!

Yield: 1 serving, with 105 calories, 6 grams fat, 2 grams protein, 18 grams carbohydrate, trace dietary fiber. That carb count looks high, I know, but the 5 grams from the Hershey's Syrup is in the form of erythritol, which is virtually unabsorbed, and 5 of the grams in the ice cream is maltitol, about half of which is absorbed. So figure about 10.5 grams net carbs—low enough for the occasional splurge.

15~Minute Snacks

Nuts and Sherry or Port

If you're not feeding children, simply passing a bowl of nuts in their shells, with nutcrackers (and plates for the shells), along with a little sherry or port, makes a nice end to a meal.

⊕ Cinnamon Splenda Nuts

This is a nice little nibble to pass around with coffee.

>2 tablespoons (28 g) butter
>
>1 cup (100 g) shelled walnuts, pecans, or a combination of the two
>
>1 1/2 to 2 tablespoons (2.3 to 3 g) Splenda
>
>1/2 teaspoon cinnamon

Melt the butter in a heavy skillet over medium heat and then add the nuts. Cook for 5 to 6 minutes, stirring from time to time. Turn off the heat, immediately sprinkle the Splenda and cinnamon over the top, and stir to distribute. (If you wait for the nuts to cool, the Splenda doesn't stick nearly so well.) I like these best warm, although they're still quite nice when cooled.

Yield: 4 or 5 servings (remember, this is just a nibble). Assuming 4 servings, each will have 5 grams of carbohydrates and 2 grams of fiber, for a total of 3 grams of usable carbs and 5 grams of protein.

☉ Candied Almonds

These are so addictive!

>1 tablespoon (14 g) butter
>
>1 cup (145) shelled almonds
>
>2 tablespoons (30 g) erythritol
>
>1 teaspoon vanilla extract
>
>1 tablespoon (1.5 g) Splenda
>
>1/2 teaspoon cinnamon

Put the butter in a Pyrex pie plate and nuke on high for 45 seconds or until melted.

Dump the almonds in the pie plate and toss with the butter until coated. Put back in the microwave and give them 2 minutes on high.

Add the erythritol and vanilla and stir to coat. Nuke another 1 minute 30 seconds and stir again. Nuke another 1 minute 30 seconds, pull them out, stir in the Splenda and cinnamon, and let them cool a few minutes, stirring now and then, before eating.

Yield: 4 servings, each with 240 calories, 21 grams fat, 7 grams protein, 8 grams carbohydrate, 4 grams dietary fiber, and 4 grams usable carb.

⊕ Roasted, Salted Pecans

You can buy cans of roasted, salted pecans, of course, but they're so much better roasted fresh in butter. They're cheaper, too.

> 1 tablespoon (14 g) butter
>
> 1 cup (100 g) pecan halves
>
> salt

Put the butter in a Pyrex pie plate and nuke on high for 30 seconds to melt. Add the pecans and toss until they're evenly coated.

Put your pecans back in the microwave and give them 90 seconds on high. Stir and give them another 90 seconds to 2 minutes. Salt and devour or keep in a snap-top container with a lid—for as long as you can resist.

Yield: 4 servings, each with 205 calories, 21 grams fat, 2 grams protein, 5 grams carbohydrate, 2 grams dietary fiber, and 3 grams usable carb.

⊕ Nacho Cheese Crisps

You've had tortilla chips with nacho cheese flavoring, no doubt. This is a big chip made of cheese with nacho flavorings. It's so much better! Do make sure your cheese has no additives—which will probably mean you'll have to shred it yourself, since most preshredded cheese has cellulose. Run it through the shredding blade of your food processor and it'll add a big 1 to 2 minutes to your recipe. Heck, even if you use your box grater you'll be done within the 15 minute time limit.

> 1 cup (115 g) shredded cheddar cheese with no additives
>
> 1/2 teaspoon garlic powder
>
> 1/2 teaspoon onion powder
>
> 1/4 teaspoon cayenne or to taste

Sprinkle the seasonings over the shredded cheese, tossing as you go.

Spray a microwaveable plate with nonstick cooking spray—I used a salad-sized plate. Put about 1/4 cup (29 g) of cheese on the plate and nuke on high for 2 to 3 minutes or until you've got a crispy disc that looks sort of like an orange surface of the moon. Let it cool a minute or two, loosen it from the surface of the plate by sliding a knife underneath, and cook another batch. I had to re-spray the plate between batches, or I got sticking.

Yield: 4 servings, each with 116 calories, 9 grams fat, 7 grams protein, 1 gram carbohydrate, and 6 grams usable carb.

⊕ Parmesan~Pine Nut~Pepper Frico

Again, you need additive-free cheese for this, and most preshredded Parmesan has cellulose in it. But I can usually find some that doesn't; I used Butoni brand, which worked great.

> 3 tablespoons (15 g) shredded Parmesan cheese—It must have no additives.
> 1/2 tablespoon pine nuts
> 1/8 teaspoon coarsely ground pepper or to taste

Spray a microwaveable plate with nonstick cooking spray. Make a low heap about 3 inches (7.5 cm) across of the Parmesan. Sprinkle the pine nuts and pepper evenly over it.

Nuke on high for 90 seconds (time may vary, depending on your microwave—this is just right in mine). Let it cool for a minute or two to crisp up and then break or cut in half and devour!

Yield: 2 servings, each with 44 calories, 3 grams fat, 3 grams protein, 1 gram carbohydrate, trace dietary fiber, and 1 gram usable carb.

☉ Cinnamon Rinds

No, I am not crazy. These are really good, especially if you're missing salty-sweet snacks like caramel corn. Be aware: Despite the slurs against them, pork rinds are very good food, far more nutritious than just about anything else in the snack aisle—look at that protein count! They're quite filling, too.

> 1 bag (5 ounces, or 140 g) pork rinds
>
> 1/4 cup (6 g) granular sucralose
>
> 1/4 teaspoon cinnamon

Yield: 5 servings, each with 160 calories, 9 grams fat, 17 grams protein, 1 gram carbohydrate, trace dietary fiber, and 1 gram usable carb.

Cheese

Cheese for dessert may sound strange to sugar-addicted Americans, but it's an old European custom. I'd never tried this until I went on the Low-Carb High Life Cruise in 2001 and discovered that Carnival Cruise Lines has cheese on the dessert menu every night. My readers and I ended up ordering a cheese platter just about every night, and we all agreed that it made a nice—and very satisfying—end to a meal. If you have any empty corners after the meal, a little cheese is guaranteed to fill them right up. It's nicest to pass a slice or two of a few varieties—perhaps some sort of blue cheese, a soft cheese such as Camembert or Brie, and a firmer cheese such as Edam or Gouda. Add some Gruyère or Havarti and perhaps a good strong cheddar, and you've got a winning assortment.

Fruit

Fruit desserts are an interesting question for the low-carb dieter. On the one hand, they're likely to have more carbohydrates than sugar-free commercially made stuff. On the other hand, they're likely to be far lower in calories—and calories still *do* count, at least some—and far, far more nutritious.

Which fruit you choose makes a big difference. A banana, for instance, will run you about 25 grams of carbohydrates, and a cup (155 g) of diced fresh pineapple has 19 grams. On the other hand, there are some fruits that are low enough in sugar to fit into our diets in moderation, and luckily for us, they're some of the most delectable. Here's a rundown of the lowest-sugar fruits, plus a few simple ideas for fruit desserts.

Apricots are a real bargain. One has just 3.9 grams of carbohydrates and 0.84 grams fiber, for a total of about 3 grams of usable carbs!

All of the berries are pretty low carb, and they make a terrific quick-and-easy dessert with either heavy cream or whipped cream. For that matter, you could eat them plain! By the way, berries are also among the most nutritious fruits available; you'll be getting a lot of benefit from the few carbs they add to your day.

- 1/2 cup (65 g) **raspberries** has 7 grams of carbohydrates and 4.2 grams of fiber, for a total of just 2.8 grams of usable carbs.

- 1/2 cup (75 g) **blackberries** has 9.2 grams of carbohydrates and 3.6 grams of fiber, for a total of 5.6 grams of usable carbs.

- 1/2 cup (75 g) **strawberries** has 5.2 grams of carbohydrates and 2 grams of fiber, for a total of 3.2 grams of usable carbs.

- 1/2 cup (75 g) **blueberries** has 10.2 grams of carbohydrates and 1.7 grams of fiber, for a total of 8.5 grams of usable carbs.

15-Minute Desserts

I didn't put in a lot of work on dessert recipes for this book for a simple reason: If you're scrambling for time and need to get everything on the table as quickly as possible, you're not going to take an extra 15 minutes to make dessert! And if you're the sort of person who simply hates cooking, you're probably going to put your limited efforts into the main meal, not the dessert.

I also live in the hope that you're working on breaking the sweet habit and are making desserts an occasional thing, rather than a daily (or even twice-daily) inevitability. That being said, you might want a little something extra at the end of your meal from time to time. Here are a few ideas for fast low-carb end-of-the-meal treats:

☺ Strawberry Crunch Parfait

In their book *The GO-Diet*, Drs. Goldberg and O'Mara explain that plain yogurt has far fewer carbs than the label would indicate because most of the lactose in the milk has been converted to lactic acid by the yogurt bacteria. Accordingly, they say that we can count just 4 grams of carbohydrates per cup (230 g) of plain yogurt. Reading this, I added yogurt back to my low-carb diet, and it's never caused weight gain or rebound hunger for me, so I think Goldberg and O'Mara are right! This recipe is so versatile—it makes a great dessert, a phenomenal quick breakfast, or a delicious and nutritious snack. Enjoy!

3 ripe strawberries

1 tablespoon (1.5 g) plus 1/4 teaspoon Splenda

3/4 cup (173 g) plain yogurt

1/2 teaspoon vanilla extract

2 tablespoons (13 g) Cinnamon Splenda Nuts, chopped a bit (see page 323)
or 2 tablespoons (16 g) Gram's Gourmet Flax 'n' Nut Crunchies (Vanilla
Almond or Cinnamon Toast flavor) or other low-carb commercial granola-
like product

Cut the green hulls off your strawberries and slice them thinly into a dish. Sprinkle
them with 1/4 teaspoon of the Splenda and stir.

Combine the yogurt with the vanilla extract and the remaining tablespoon (1.5 g) of
Splenda, stirring well. Spoon over the strawberries. Top with the nuts or Flax 'n' Nut
Crunchies and devour!

Yield: 1 serving. Using the *GO-Diet's* carb count of 4 grams of carbohydrates per cup
(230 g) of plain yogurt, this has 12 grams of carbohydrates and 3 grams of fiber, for a
total of 9 grams of usable carbs and 10 grams of protein.

Note: Feel free to substitute 1/4 cup (36 g) blueberries, (36 g) blackberries, or
(31 g) raspberries, or even (43 g) diced peaches. Make this in a clear glass dish, or
even layer it in a parfait glass, and it'll look pretty enough for company.

⊕ Fast Strawberry-Orange Sauce

This is especially nice for spiffing up a simple dessert for company, using up strawberries threatening to go bad in the refrigerator, or just because it's Tuesday.

>   1/2 cup strawberries—(73 g) fresh, or (123 g) frozen with no sugar added, thawed
>   1 tablespoon (1.5 g) Splenda
>   1/4 teaspoon orange extract

Assemble the ingredients in a food processor and purée. Serve over sliced melon or sugar-free ice cream or stir it into plain yogurt.

Yield: About 1/3 cup (85 g), or 3 servings, each with 2 grams of carbohydrates and 1 gram of fiber, for a total of 1 gram of usable carbs and a trace of protein.

⊕ Strawberry Ice Cream

Wow. All I can say is just wow. If you only try one dessert recipe from this book, make it this one.

>   1 pound (455 g) frozen unsweetened strawberries
>   1 1/2 cups (355 ml) heavy cream
>   1/4 cup (6 g) Splenda
>   1/2 tablespoon lemon juice

Put everything in your food processor and run it until the strawberries are ground up. This may require prying a strawberry off the blade a few times! The strawberries freeze the cream, and you get really, truly ice cream with an insanely great strawberry flavor. Keep in mind that if you have some left over, you can store it in a snap-top container in the freezer, but because of the lack of sugar it will freeze rock-hard. Take it out of the freezer a good half an hour before you want to eat it to let it soften a bit.

Yield: 6 servings, each with 236 calories, 22 grams fat, 2 grams protein, 10 grams carbohydrate, 2 grams dietary fiber, and 8 grams usable carb.

⊕ 5 Minute Chocolate Mug Cake

This is my de-carbed version of a recipe that's been going around the internet. You are now never more than five minutes from low carb chocolate cake; use this power responsibly! By the way, this has enough protein to make a good breakfast, and it's quick enough for a school morning. And you thought you couldn't get your kids to eat a good breakfast.

3 tablespoons (45 ml) coconut oil

2 tablespoons (14 g) almond meal

2 tablespoons (16 g) vanilla whey protein powder

3 tablespoons (45 g) erythritol

1 tablespoon (5 g) cocoa powder

1 pinch salt

1/8 teaspoon baking powder

1 egg

3 tablespoons (45 ml) half and half

Put the coconut oil in a big coffee mug you've coated with nonstick cooking spray and nuke it just until the oil is melted—maybe 30 seconds at 60% power. You just want it liquid, not hot enough to cook everything else.

Remove the mug from the microwave and measure everything else into it. Use a smallish whisk to mix it up until the batter is smooth—be sure there are no pockets of dry stuff anywhere and that it's all well-blended.

Put it back in the microwave and cook for three minutes on full power. It'll rise above the edge of the mug but should be solid enough not to spill.

When the three minutes are up, pull it out, let it cool a few minutes, tip out on a plate, cut in two, and enjoy.

Whipped cream or sugar-free vanilla ice cream would be nice with this, but we ate it as-is, and it was moist and yummy.

Yield: 2 servings, each with 335 calories, 28 grams fat, 18 grams protein, 6 grams carbohydrate, and 12 grams usable carb.

⊕ 5 Minute Gingerbread Mug Pudding

Having made the *5 Minute Chocolate Mug Cake,* I thought I'd try gingerbread. It came out quite moist, more like a steamed pudding than a cake, but I rather liked it that way, and the flavor was great. So here it is.

- 3 tablespoons (45 ml) coconut oil
- 2 tablespoons (14 g) almond meal
- 2 tablespoons (16 g) vanilla whey protein powder
- 2 tablespoons (30 g) erythritol
- 2 tablespoons (3 g) Splenda
- 1 pinch salt
- 1/8 teaspoon baking powder
- 1 teaspoon ground cinnamon
- 1 teaspoon ground ginger
- 1 pinch ground cloves
- 1 pinch ground nutmeg
- 3 tablespoons (45 ml) half and half
- 1 egg

Put the coconut oil in a big coffee mug you've coated with nonstick cooking spray and nuke it just until the oil is melted—maybe 30 seconds at 60% power. You just want it liquid, not hot enough to cook everything else.

Remove the mug from the microwave and measure everything else into it. Use a smallish whisk to mix it up until the batter is smooth—be sure there are no pockets of dry stuff anywhere and that it's all well-blended.

Put it back in the microwave and cook for three minutes on full power. It'll rise above the edge of the mug but should be solid enough not to spill.

When the three minutes are up, pull it out, let it cool a few minutes, tip out on a plate, cut in two, and enjoy.

This is even yummier with a scoop of sugar-free vanilla ice cream. Just try feeling sorry for yourself!

Yield: 2 servings, each with 342 calories, 28 grams fat, 18 grams protein, 8 grams carbohydrate, 1 gram dietary fiber, and 7 grams usable carb.

☺ Figs with Gorgonzola

It doesn't get any simpler or more elegant than this.

> 4 fresh, medium figs
>
> 1/4 cup (30 g) crumbled Gorgonzola cheese
>
> 1/2 cup (40 g) chopped walnuts

Slice the figs in half, spread each half with a tablespoon (8 g) of Gorgonzola, and sprinkle with 1/2 tablespoon chopped walnuts.

Yield: 4 servings of 2 halves, each with 12 grams of carbohydrates and 2 grams of fiber, for a total of 10 grams of usable carbs and 9 grams of protein.

Note: Some people like to broil the figs for a few minutes first.

I adore **pink grapefruit**, and since I've gone low-carb, it tastes really sweet to me! Grapefruit is higher in carbs than berries are but still pretty okay: 1/2 medium grapefruit has 10.4 grams of carbohydrates and 1.4 grams of fiber, for a total of 9 grams of usable carbs. If you'd like to spiff up that grapefruit a little, you could sprinkle it with Splenda, or as many people have suggested to me, Brown Sugar Twin. Personally, I drizzle my grapefruit with 1/4 teaspoon blackstrap molasses, which adds 1 scant gram of carbohydrates. I love the warm brown flavor of the molasses contrasted with the cool, sharp flavor of the grapefruit.

☺ Broiled Grapefruit

This is a classic sort of recipe.

> 1/2 grapefruit
>
> 1/2 teaspoon butter (optional)
>
> Splenda
>
> A touch of blackstrap molasses, if you like
>
> Ground cinnamon (optional)

Loosen the sections of the grapefruit by running a sharp, thin-bladed knife around each one. Sprinkle with the sweetener of your choice, plus cinnamon if you like, and broil a few inches (7.5 to 10 cm) from the flame for 10 minutes.

Yield: 1 serving, with 10.4 grams of carbohydrates and 1.4 grams of fiber, for a total of 9 grams of usable carbs from the grapefruit. Splenda has 0.5 grams of carbohydrates per teaspoon. Blackstrap has 1 gram of carbohydrates per 1/4 teaspoon—and it's so strong-flavored you won't want to use more than this!

Note: Some people like to cut the white core out and put butter in there.

Melon is a great low-carb dessert, and it's very nutritious. If you'd like to fancy it up a bit, sprinkle it with a little lime juice mixed with Splenda and ginger to taste or top it with the *Fast Strawberry Orange Sauce* (see page 331)—but it's really a fine dessert as-is.

- 1/8 of a medium **cantaloupe** has 8.4 grams of carbohydrates and 0.8 grams of fiber, for a total of 7.6 grams of usable carbs.

- 1/8 of a medium **honeydew** has 9.2 grams of carbohydrates and 0.6 grams of fiber, for a total of 8.6 grams of usable carbs.

- 1 cup (173 g) of frozen **melon balls** has 8 grams of carbohydrates and 0.7 grams of fiber, for a total of 7.3 grams of usable carbs.

- 1 cup (150 g) diced **watermelon** has 11 grams of carbohydrates and 0.8 grams of fiber, for a total of 10.2 grams of usable carbs.

- One medium-size **nectarine** has 11.8 grams of carbohydrates and 1.6 grams of fiber, for a total of 10.2 grams of usable carbs.

- One medium **peach** has 11.1 grams of carbohydrates and 2 grams of fiber, for a total of 9.1 grams of usable carbs.

- One medium **plum** has 13.1 grams of carbohydrates and 1.5 grams of fiber, for a total of 11.6 grams of usable carbs.

- 1 medium fresh **fig** has 9.6 grams of carbohydrates and 1.6 grams of fiber, for a total of 8 grams of usable carbs.

☉ Speedy Low-Carb Peach Melba

This is a short-cut, no-sugar-added version of a very famous dessert—and it's scrumptious! You can use fresh peaches in this, if you'd prefer, but unlike the frozen ones, you'll have to peel and slice them, which may take you over the 15-minute time limit.

> 2 cups (500 g) frozen, sliced, no-sugar-added peaches
> 1/4 cup (60 ml) lemon juice
> 1/4 teaspoon orange extract
> 1/2 cup (12 g) Splenda
> 1 cup raspberries—(125 g) fresh or (250 g) frozen with no sugar added
> 4 tablespoons (28 g) toasted slivered almonds (optional)

Don't bother to thaw the frozen peaches. Put them in a microwaveable bowl, mix together 2 tablespoons (28 ml) of the lemon juice, the orange extract, and half of the Splenda, and pour it over them. Cover (I just lay a plate on top) and microwave on High for 5 to 7 minutes or until tender right through.

While the peaches are poaching, put the raspberries, the remaining 2 tablespoons (28 ml) of lemon juice, and the remaining Splenda in your food processor with the S-blade in place. Pulse a few times until everything is puréed together.

When the peaches are done, divide between 4 small serving dishes and divide the raspberry sauce between them. Sprinkle each dish with a tablespoon (7 g) of almonds, if desired. Serve.

Yield: 4 servings, each with 17 grams of carbohydrates and 4 grams of fiber, for a total of 13 grams of usable carbs and 1 gram of protein. Add the optional almonds and each serving has 19 grams of carbohydrates and 5 grams of fiber, for a total of 14 grams of usable carbs and 3 grams of protein.

✫ This also has a mere 68 calories, every one of them nutritious.

Note: Now, this is not the traditional way to serve Peach Melba—the traditional way would include a scoop of vanilla ice cream. You could do this, of course, using one of the no-sugar-added ice creams, but since this is already in the upper range of the low-carb recipe spectrum, I'd probably only do this for a very special occasion. You could also serve this with vanilla yogurt—see the *Strawberry Crunch Parfait* recipe (see page 329) for how-tos—and add only about 2.5 grams of carbs per 1/2 cup (115 g) of yogurt.

> **Tip:** Feel free to make the raspberry sauce all by itself—it's great over melon, stirred into plain yogurt, or as an elegant quick dessert when combined with no-sugar ice cream.

Purchased Low-Carb Sweets

Low-carbohydrate chocolate or other sugar-free candy. This stuff gets better all the time and is now widely available. Since sugar-free candy is polyol-sweetened, it does technically have carbs in it, but the amount that most of you will absorb will be quite low. Still, both because of the possibility of more carb absorption than the labels let on and because of possible gastric distress, go easy, okay? My husband and I will often split a 1.5 ounce (43 g) sugar-free dark chocolate bar for dessert; this strikes me as plenty.

Sugar-free cocoa, made from mix. Read the labels on all the brands available at your grocery store—in mine, Swiss Miss Diet is the lowest in carbs, at 4 grams per cup (235 ml).

No-Sugar-Added Ice Cream. The no-sugar ice cream is pretty darned good. My favorite is the brand called Dreyer's in the West and Edy's in the East, but Breyer's also makes one, and my grocery store even has a house brand of no-sugar-added ice cream. This stuff does still have usable, absorbable carbs in it—the lactose in the milk it was made from—so go *easy*. A "serving" is 1/2 cup (70 g), not a half a carton! The carb counts vary some, so *read your labels*.

No-Sugar-Added Ice Pops. The Popsicle company makes a sugar-free variety, and they're among your lowest-carb prepared desserts—just 3 grams per pop and only 15 calories. So if you're a Popsicle fan, your dessert problems are solved! They're available in two assortments, either orange, cherry, and grape or the new tropical flavors, Caribbean fruit punch, Hawaiian pineapple, and tropical orange.

No-Sugar-Added Fudge Pops. No-sugar-added Fudgsicles taste just like the Fudgsicles of your youth—really, they do. Looking at the Popsicle company Website, they say these have 19 grams of carbohydrates and 1 gram of fiber per serving, which sounds like you're going to get a prohibitive 18 grams of carbs. But 3 grams are "sugar alcohols," aka polyols, so you can subtract them out, too, leaving 15 grams. Then you take a look at the "serving size"—which is two pops, not one. So if you eat one pop—which is what I'd be likely to do—you'll get 7.5 grams of usable carbs. And *that* fits into your low-carb diet!

There are also store brands of sugar-free fudge pops around; I know that Kroger—the biggest grocery chain in the United States—has one. Make sure to read the labels to find the true usable carb count and don't forget to look at the serving size.

Sugar-Free Gelatin. It takes more than 15 minutes to make gelatin, if you count the chilling time, but Jell-O, for one, makes prepared sugar-free gelatin in plastic cups with peel-off tops; look for them under the name "Jell-O Snacks." If you like gelatin, this could be a handy item to keep in the pantry.

Sugar-Free Instant Pudding. Mix this with half heavy cream, half water to eliminate half of the carbs that using milk would add. If you do this before sitting down to dinner and set it in the refrigerator to chill, it should be at least passably thickened by the time dessert rolls around. According to my calculations, using the sugar-free instant pudding I have in the pantry, this would come to 8 grams of carbohydrates per serving.

15~Minute Smoothies

Smoothies are hugely popular, super-quick both to make and to consume, and it's easy to load in a meal's worth of protein. I wrote a smoothies book, but sadly several of the ingredients I used most in that book have since disappeared from most markets. So I thought it would be nice to include a selection of smoothies in this book. One of my best discoveries in recent years has been that cottage cheese makes great, creamy low carb smoothies, so I've included it in several of these recipes.

⊕ Mexican Chocolate Smoothie

This is far and away my favorite smoothie I came up with for this book. The combination of chocolate, vanilla, and cinnamon is classically Mexican and enchanting. Try this!

> 3/4 cup (165 g) cottage cheese
>
> 1/4 cup (80 g) sugar-free vanilla coffee flavoring syrup
>
> 1/4 cup (60 ml) water
>
> 1/4 cup (32 g) vanilla whey protein powder
>
> 1 tablespoon (6 g) cocoa powder
>
> 1/4 teaspoon cinnamon
>
> 4 ice cubes
>
> 1 teaspoon guar, xanthan, or glucomannan or to taste

Throw everything from the cottage cheese through the cinnamon in your blender and start it running. Add the ice cubes one by one, waiting until one is ground up before adding the next. When all the ice is in, thicken to taste with guar, xanthan, or glucomannan—I used 1 teaspoon of glucomannan, and it was perfect.

Yield: 1 serving, with 388 calories, 8 grams fat, 67 grams protein, 14 grams carbohydrate, 4 grams dietary fiber, and 10 grams usable carb.

⊕ Almond Joy Smoothie

I wanted a smoothie recipe using coconut milk, and I had just gotten the Almond Roca syrup, so you see what the result was.

> 3/4 cup (175 ml) unsweetened coconut milk
>
> 1/4 cup (60 g) sugar-free Almond Roca syrup
>
> 2 tablespoons (12 g) cocoa powder
>
> 5 drops coconut extract
>
> 1 teaspoon guar, xanthan, or glucomannan, or to taste
>
> 1/4 cup (32 g) vanilla whey protein powder
>
> 4 ice cubes

Just assemble everything but the ice in your blender and run. Drop in the ice cubes one at a time and continue blending until the ice is pulverized. Pour into a glass and drink.

Yield: 1 serving, with 248 calories, 5 grams fat, 45 grams protein, 11 grams carbohydrate, 5 grams dietary fiber, and 6 grams usable carb.

⊕ Mounds Smoothie

   3/4 cup (175 ml) unsweetened coconut milk

   1/4 cup (60 g) sugar-free chocolate coffee flavoring syrup

   2 tablespoons (12 g) cocoa powder

   5 drops coconut flavoring (find this in the baking aisle, near the vanilla
      extract)

   1/4 cup (32 g) vanilla whey protein powder

   4 ice cubes

   glucomannan

Just assemble everything but the ice in your blender and run. Drop in the ice cubes one at a time and continue blending until the ice is pulverized. Pour into a glass and drink.

Yield: 1 serving, with 248 calories, 5 grams fat, 45 grams protein, 11 grams carbohydrate, 5 grams dietary fiber, and 6 grams usable fiber.

⊕ Snickers Smoothie

This smoothie has chocolate, caramel, and peanut, just like a Snickers bar!

   3/4 cup (165 g) cottage cheese

   2 tablespoons (28 g) chocolate sugar-free coffee flavoring syrup

   2 tablespoons (28 g) caramel sugar-free coffee flavoring syrup

   1 tablespoon (6 g) cocoa powder

   2 tablespoons (32 g) natural peanut butter

   1 tablespoon (8 g) vanilla whey protein powder

   1/4 cup (60 ml) water

   4 ice cubes

   1/2 teaspoon guar, xanthan, or glucomannan, or to taste

Throw everything but the ice and thickener in your blender and start it running. Add the ice a cube at a time and then thicken to taste.

Yield: 1 serving, with 405 calories, 20 grams fat, 42 grams protein, 17 grams carbohydrate, 4 grams dietary fiber, and 13 grams usable carb.

⊕ Almond Roca Smoothie

I thought of this the second I saw sugar-free Almond Roca syrup sitting on the shelf.

3/4 cup (165 g) cottage cheese

2 tablespoons (32 g) almond butter

2 tablespoons (28 g) sugar-free Almond Roca coffee flavoring syrup

2 tablespoons (28 g) chocolate sugar-free coffee flavoring syrup

2 tablespoons (16 g) vanilla whey protein powder

1 tablespoon (6 g) cocoa powder

4 ice cubes

3/4 teaspoon guar, xanthan, or glucomannan or to taste

Throw everything but the ice and thickener in your blender and start it running. Add the ice a cube at a time and then thicken to taste.

Yield: 1 serving, with 473 calories, 24 grams fat, 51 grams protein, 18 grams carbohydrate, 4 grams dietary fiber, and 14 grams usable carb.

☺ Super Strawberry Smoothie

The strawberries make this a little higher carb than some smoothies, but they're awfully nutritious.

  3/4 cup (165 g) cottage cheese

  1/2 cup (128 g) frozen strawberries, unsweetened

  1/4 cup (60 g) sugar-free strawberry syrup

  1/4 cup (60 ml) water

  4 ice cubes

  1 teaspoon lemon juice

  1/4 cup (32 g) vanilla whey protein powder

Throw everything but the ice and thickener in your blender and start it running. Add the ice a cube at a time, waiting until one is pulverized before you add the next. When all the ice is in, it's done!

Yield: 1 serving, with 402 calories, 7 grams fat, 67 grams protein, 18 grams carbohydrate, 3 grams dietary fiber, and 15 grams usable carb.

☺ Peach-Strawberry Smoothie

This has such a gorgeous color! It tastes great, too. It's also higher carb than some of the other smoothies, though, because of the fruit, so let your own personal body be your guide.

  1 cup (230 g) plain yogurt

  5 frozen unsweetened strawberries

  1/2 cup (125 g) frozen unsweetened sliced peaches

  1/4 cup (32 g) vanilla whey protein powder

  8 teaspoons (4 g) Splenda, or the equivalent in liquid Splenda

  1/2 teaspoon guar, xanthan, or glucomannan or to taste

Just put everything in your blender and run until it's smooth.

Yield: 1 serving, with 427 calories, 12 grams fat, 53 grams protein, 23 grams carbohydrate, 5 grams dietary fiber, and 18 grams usable carb.

⊕ Peaches and Cream Smoothie

This makes a great breakfast on a hot summer morning.

> 3/4 cup (165 g) cottage cheese
>
> 1/3 cup (83 g) sugar-free frozen peach slices
>
> 1/4 cup (60 g) sugar-free peach flavored syrup
>
> 1/4 cup (60 ml) water
>
> 1/4 cup (32 g) vanilla whey protein powder
>
> 1 teaspoon lemon juice
>
> 4 ice cubes
>
> 1 teaspoon guar, xanthan, or glucomannan or to taste

Throw everything but the ice and thickener in your blender and start it running. Add the ice a cube at a time and then thicken to taste—1 teaspoon glucomannan was about right for me.

Yield: 1 serving, with 399 calories, 7 grams fat, 67 grams protein, 18 grams carbohydrate, 3 grams dietary fiber, and 15 grams usable carb.

Note: I use unsweetened frozen peach slices. Let them partially thaw the first time and see how many pack into your 1/3 cup (60 ml) measuring cup. After that, you can just count out that many slices instead of having to dirty up a measuring cup. Plus, that way you can put them in the blender still frozen.

15-Minute "Cereal"

Okay, so this has its own chapter because it doesn't fit in with anything else. But it's a great recipe, and I think a lot of people will find it useful, so it deserves its own chapter!

⊕ Almond-Coconut Hot Cereal

I've heard from many people who long for hot cereal on cold mornings. Here's a fast, creamy, and very filling breakfast for all you oatmeal-lovers. It has more protein than three eggs and far more fiber than oatmeal.

> 2 tablespoons (14 g) almond meal
> 2 tablespoons (14 g) flax seed meal
> 1 tablespoon (8 g) vanilla whey protein powder
> 1 tablespoon (5 g) finely shredded coconut meat
> 1 pinch salt
> 1 tablespoon (15 g) almond butter
> 1/3 cup (80 ml) boiling water

Spoon the almond meal, flax seed meal, vanilla whey protein, coconut, and salt into a bowl and stir together. Add the almond butter and pour in the boiling water. Stir until the almond butter is melted in. Serve with cream or half and half and sweetener of your choice.

Yield: 1 serving, with 379 calories, 25 grams fat, 27 grams protein, 19 grams carbohydrate, 10 grams dietary fiber, and 9 grams usable carb.

Note: To streamline this even further, mix together 12 tablespoons (84 g) each of almond meal and flax seed meal and 6 tablespoons each of vanilla whey protein (48 g) and shredded coconut (30 g) and keep in a snap-top container—this is six servings worth. To make cereal, put 1/3 cup (37 g) of this mixture in a bowl with a pinch of salt and a tablespoon (7 g) of almond butter and add 1/3 cup (80 ml) boiling water.

About the Author

DANA CARPENDER is a best-selling author and radio host who was startled to discover that limiting her carbohydrate intake not only helped her control her weight, but also produced the health and vitality a low-fat diet had promised but never delivered. More than fifteen years later, she laughs at people who say "You can't eat that way long-term." Her nine cookbooks are the result of her realization that the key to permanent dietary change is the answer to the age-old question, "What's for supper?" To date they have sold over a million copies worldwide. Dana blogs about low-carb nutrition at www.HoldtheToast.com; her weekly blog digest goes out to over 20,000 readers. She is also managing editor of *CarbSmart Magazine* at www.CarbSmart.com, as well as a featured staff writer. She launched her internet radio show and podcast, Dana's Low Carb For Life, in January 2011. Dana lives in Bloomington, Indiana, with her husband and a menagerie of pets, all of whom are well and healthily fed.

Index